The Spirit of the Hedgerow

The Spirit
of the Hedgerow

JO DUNBAR

WINNER OF THE LOCAL LEGEND
SPIRITUAL WRITING COMPETITION

A record of this publication is available from the British Library.

ISBN 978-1-910027-16-5

Typesetting by Wordzworth Ltd
www.wordzworth.com

Cover design by Titanium Design Ltd
www.titaniumdesign.co.uk

Cover and body painting images © WildWays Body Painting Project

All other images © the Author

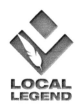

Published by Local Legend
www.local-legend.co.uk

LOCAL
LEGEND

Dedicated to the Goddess and the Green Man of the land,
and to the plants of the hedgerows in all their manifest
and unmanifest forms.

www.local-legend.co.uk

About this Book

Since the beginning of human history, our ancestral roots and those of the hedgerows have been intimately entangled. Now, often forgotten amongst the hedgerows, the 'wild weeds' still offer amazing medicinal opportunities, delicious sources of food and fascinating legends of our past. Many of the secrets of our history lie hidden in the stories of these plants. Our ancestors, living in harmony with the cycles of nature, knew how to prepare wild food, prepare remedies, make protective talismans and so much more. But we have lost our connection with the magic of nature...

In this fascinating and unique book, richly illustrated, Jo Dunbar shows us what we so often miss in the beauty all around us. We learn here which plants to pick (or avoid!) and how to use them for ourselves. And woven in with this are the ancient stories and folklore of the countryside, firing our imagination and helping us to communicate in a real way with our natural environment.

This book is the winner of the Local Legend Spiritual Writing Competition.

About the Author

Jo Dunbar has been practising as a medical herbalist since 1999 and is the founder of Botanica Medica herbal apothecary. It was through growing and collecting the herbs for her apothecaries that she developed a personal relationship with hedgerow plants and trees. This love of nature led her also to follow the Druidic path, honouring all lifeforms on Earth as well as the cycles of the year. Woven in with this are the ancient stories and the folklore of the countryside, firing our imagination and helping us to communicate in a real way with our cousins in nature.

Jo grew up in South Africa where she first studied horticulture and worked with Xhosa men who taught her about indigenous plants and how they are used magically and medically. She now lives in Hampshire, England.

www.jodunbar.co.uk
www.botanicamedica.co.uk

Previous Publications

How to Cope Successfully with Candida (Wellhouse Publishing Ltd, 2003)
Recovering from Stress, Burn Out and Fatigue (self-published)

Contents

Our Ancient Roots

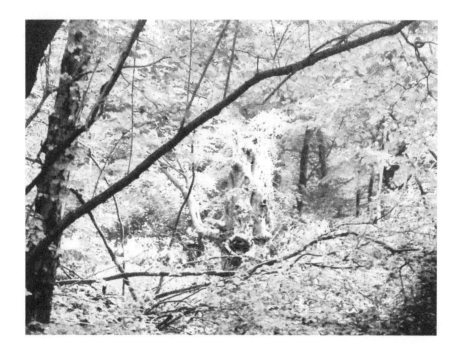

Since the beginning of human history, our ancestral roots and those of the hedgerows have been intimately entangled. Now, often forgotten amongst the hedgerows, the 'wild weeds' still offer amazing medicinal opportunities, delicious sources of food and fascinating folklore from our past. Many of the secrets of our history lie hidden in the stories of these plants. Our ancestors, living in harmony with the cycles of nature, knew how to prepare wild food and remedies, make protective talismans and so much more. But we have lost our connection with the magic of nature, and are much the poorer for it.

During the Celtic and Anglo-Saxon periods in Britain, large areas of ancient woodland were cleared for agriculture and animal grazing.

I

Small clans of people lived at the forest's edge, in homes made from mud, wattle and thatch. By cutting back the forest, the regrowth would have produced a rough hedge and inside this would be a clearing that represented domesticity, order and safety. On the other side of the hedge, within the dark forest, lurked fearsome bears, wolves, wild boar, serpents and also dragons, elves and 'the other folk'.

A highlight during the cycles of the seasons was the visiting bards, with songs of legends and stories from faraway places. Many times these myth-spinners were also healers and their visit would include tending a sickly person or an unproductive field where they worked their magic using incantations and herbs.

After the chores of the day were done, the people would gather in the flickering firelight of their mead halls to listen to the storyteller recount long tales of warriors and heroes, kings, dragons and elves. Perhaps outside the thin walls, the winds would scream and wolves would howl. In those days, the nights were very dark with only the bright moon and sharp stars for light. Sounds were louder, shadows deeper, and images might be glimpsed in the fiery shadows, especially when minds were softened with mead and ale, and the perils of the forest were very close.

Giants and dragons were real to these folk – after all, everyone had seen the firedrakes flying across the starry skies from time to time. Today, we call them comets. Certain wells or pits were known to be the lairs of these fearful dragon worms, or 'wyrms'. Even today, some places still hold names such as Dragon Hill at Uffington where there is some debate as to whether the ancient chalk engraving into the hill represents a dragon rather than a stylised white horse.

The collective mindset was animistic and magical. In the Celtic and Anglo-Saxon eras and beyond, people believed in faeries and elves. These were not the small winged creatures of our Victorian fairy tales, but a race that lived alongside ours yet for the most part remained unseen. Elf beings could be smaller than us or taller, and they might be as likely to bestow favours and comfort on a homestead as to cause terrible mischief, so they had to be constantly placated. Certainly they were never referred to as fairies, which was considered rude, but rather they were known as 'the fair folk', 'the good folk', 'the little people' or 'the gentry' and, even up until the last century, faery folk were sturdily believed in by country folk, particularly of the western counties of Britain.

Something greatly feared by the Anglo-Saxons was 'elf shot', experienced as a sudden and unexpected sharp pain such as hiccups or, more severely, a difficulty in breathing with sharp pains in the chest. In these cases it was likely that malicious elves had shot invisible arrows into their victim, allowing the life force to leak out, sometimes to the extent that the victim died. Today we would probably diagnose those symptoms as pleurisy. The Anglo-Saxons cured elf shot with a plant called elf-wort, now known as *Inula helenium*; modern medical herbalists use the same plant to treat pleurisy. The same disease and the same plant, just a completely different cultural understanding.

Having said that, it is not so very different because science tells us that tiny creatures invisible to the naked eye (bacteria or viruses) do invade our bodies and cause illnesses such as pleurisy. We now understand the plant to have antibacterial properties and we have the scientific evidence; but then the Anglo-Saxons also had their own evidence, in the form of elven (Neolithic) arrowheads which they turned up when cultivating the soil.

In those ancient times, disease and discontent was said to be caused by magic and plants were used to combat this dark magic. Not only did the plants of the hedgerow protect by forming a physical barrier against the dark forest, but they were also used as antidotes to malevolent magic. The Celtic, Anglo-Saxon and medieval folk had relationships with plants in a way that is very rare these days. Having an animistic consciousness, they believed that all natural things, such as plants, animals, mountains and rivers, have a spirit or a life force, and this can influence human events.

3

The magic and power of herbs occurred when the wizards of ancient times invoked the life force of the plant to heal the life force of the unwell human or animal. When a person became ill, they had somehow lost some of their life force, either through elf arrows, flying venoms or injury. Today, when we are ill, we too feel fatigued, with weak muscles and a difficulty in thinking clearly. Sometimes we recover spontaneously and sometimes we call upon herbs to restore our health so that we once again feel hale and hearty. Although there are many biological constituents in plants, there is that inexplicable extra dimension that herbalists secretly call 'the magic', which supports the healing process so naturally and comfortably!

Hedgerow plants were thought to be imbued with benevolent magical properties and because of this they were deeply respected. The herbs were seen as powerful beings, to be honoured and harvested with great care and dedication. Today, most people despise these same plants as 'weeds' because we have been brainwashed into disenchantment with the natural world, but I am inviting you to re-enchant your life by remembering our ancient animistic consciousness and the magic of the hedgerow: that is, re-membering, becoming once again a member of the magical world of nature.

We can reunite our lives with the wild plants in the hedgerows by following the year as it gently spins its seasonal cycles. As a medical herbalist who harvests much of her medicines from the hedgerows, I have watched the various plants in the hedges blossom, fruit and decay at certain times of the year, and taken note of their stories and properties. In doing so, I have come to regard the hedgerow as a natural clock, in that I can tell where I am in 'the herbal year' by looking at which plants are currently showing off in the hedges. So I plot my herbalist's life according to the hedgerow clock.

This book tells some of the stories and uses of these special plants in a way that I feel the plants would like their stories to be told. You will meet the plants as personalities rather than just as botanical species with medical properties. It is so easy to fall in love with the wild magic of these plants that weave their way through the hedgerows across these isles.

As you wander along the hedgerows, I do hope to remind you of the wonderful allies that we have in these 'weeds', and to engender in you a feeling of kindliness towards our natural healing plants. You might even develop a bond of friendship with certain plants. This is not weird – humans have been doing this for millions of years. We have only recently forgotten.

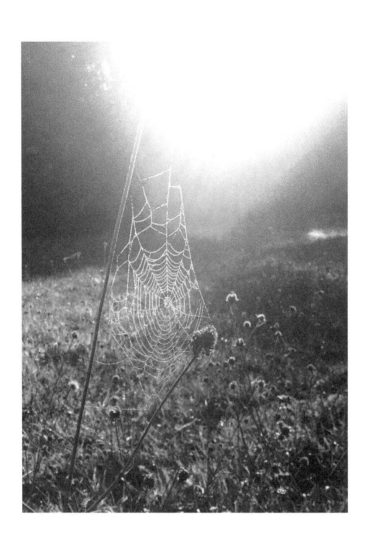

The Wheel of the Year

In ancient days, people were very observant of the seasons because they were usually either nomadic foragers or farming folk and their livelihood depended on planting and harvesting. They also appear to have been very concerned with matters of life, death and fertility, and with propitiating the gods with ceremony and gifts to ensure favourable outcomes for their harvest. Thus, they noticed the longest day and shortest day of the year, the dates when night and day were of equal length, and they also celebrated the cross-quarter days. These ceremonies may not all have been celebrated as an annual cycle, but Neo-Pagans today honour all eight celebrations of the Wheel of the Year. It is nice to know about them, because we can link our lives to these regular celebrations, which occur approximately every six weeks throughout the year. We can even personalise these celebrations, for example, by holding a small ceremony of gratitude at harvest time or of remembrance of Granny at Samhain (Hallowe'en).

There is some indecision as to when exactly the Celtic year began, so I am going to begin our tour of the hedgerow year with the first signs of spring, celebrated in very early February with Imbolc.

The Eight Celebrations of the Celtic Year

2nd February *   Imbolc: a fire festival as the first green shoots appear after the long dark days of winter.

21st March   The spring equinox: a solar festival midway between the winter and summer solstices. Days and nights are now of equal length, with the light becoming the dominant force.

1st May   Beltane: a fire festival and May Day, celebrating the union of the god and the goddess and the fertility of the land.

21st June   The summer solstice: a solar festival and the longest day of the year.

1st August   Lughnasadh: a fire festival of thanksgiving for the first harvest.

21st September   The autumn equinox: a solar festival midway between the summer and winter solstices. Nights and days are of equal length with the dark becoming the dominant force.

31st October   Samhain: a fire festival. This is the night when the veil between this world and 'the other world' is thinnest so there may be communication with the ancestors.

21st December   The winter solstice or Yule: a solar festival and the shortest day of the year.

* the dates given above are traditional and can vary slightly in modern times

February

It is the time of Imbolc. Before the industrial revolution, when most people lived off the land, it was not always a reliable probability that they would survive the winter. The damp, cold, scarcity of food and contagion made winters very hard. Many died. Even now, it is with relief that we see the first signs of new life in early February. Imbolc means 'in milk'. The ewes have not yet lambed but they soon will.

Small green shoots peep out of the frosty earth and give hope for the passing of winter into spring. We look forward joyously toward the warmth of sun. At this time of the year it is pale and weak, yet the light is growing and the sun will gather strength. Seeds are germinating just under the earth so this is the time for the renewal of life, of hope and of new beginnings.

Bullace, Wild Plum (*Prunus insititia*) and Sloe, Blackthorn (*Prunus spinosa*)

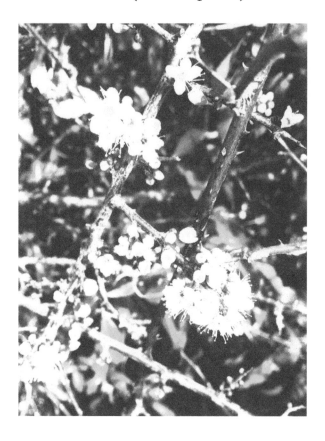

One of the country names for blackthorn (the sloe tree) is 'Snow in Spring', being one of the first trees to flower in the spring, covering patches of hedgerow in small white blossoms and heralding the promise of brighter, warmer days. At last, life begins to stir in the hedges. Yet this plant also carries a rather dark reputation in country lore, which may have developed because a puncture from its thorn feels so evil. Accompanied by great pain, the wound often becomes septic and can spread to create reactive arthritis in remote parts of the body. The venomous nature of the wound was the reason why dark witches used the thorns to pierce wax poppets in their spells of evil intention.

The Irish believed that the blackthorn was protected by faeries unfriendly to humans. Some say that the tree demands a blood sacrifice and a friend of mine who cuts small branches to carve wands from tells me that he never comes away without being bloodied from a scratch or puncture wound.

The ancient Celtic Ogham (tree oracle) associates the plant with harsh challenges, or fate that cannot be avoided. Blackthorn is associated with darkness, strife and evil intentions that are destructive, ruinous and cannot be side-stepped. Although blackthorn has been used in black magic to create mayhem in people's lives, by the same token it can be used to protect during times of chaos. Its powerful energy will create a strong and impenetrable hedge around you, protecting against evil influences.

On a much lighter note, both the sloe and the wild damson (bullace) are included together here as their medical uses are the same, but their culinary delights are wildly different. I discovered that I have a wild damson tree in the hedgerow bordering my garden, a delightful tree. The rosy petals whirling softly down to the lawn is like snow in springtime. One of my favourite ways of passing time in April is to lie underneath the tree listening to the birds singing whilst watching petals fluttering through the bright blue sky. In the late summer, it is a joy to stand under the tree, enjoying the sweet plump fruit fresh off the arching branches.

Despite my greed, I have never got the expected diarrhoea from eating too much fresh fruit, and that would be because both sloes and bullace fruit have a binding action and can actually be used for the treatment of diarrhoea. The flowers of both plants, on the other hand, act as a mild laxative. To achieve this, make an infusion and sweeten it with honey – a rather nice cleanser. So we see that these two plants both loosen the bowels and restrict diarrhoea, depending on which part of the plant you use.

We all know about sloe gin, which is very easily made. Damsons make excellent jam with apples or, when stewed with brown sugar and cinnamon, can be enjoyed with live plain yoghurt as a healthy dessert.

Bullace and Apple Cheese

I kg windfall apples
I cup of water
I kg of bullaces
Sugar

Cut out and discard bruised parts of the apples, then cut the apples but do not peel or core them. Put them into a preserving pan with the water and simmer until soft. Add the sloes or bullace fruit and continue simmering until they too are soft. Rub the fruit through a sieve then weigh the fruit puree, returning it to the pan with an equal weight of sugar. Stir over a low heat until the sugar has dissolved, bring to a boil and then simmer, stirring all the time until the mixture is thick. This takes about an hour. Pour the mixture into sterilised jars, seal them and allow all to set. It adds an interesting dimension to drop a generous sprig of thyme into each jar to bring a herby sweetness to the fruit cheese. This is delicious with strong cheese on an oat biscuit, or herb pork or venison sausages.

Lichen (*Usnea species*)

A long time ago, a friend asked me what the ancient Britons had used as an antibiotic agent when they were cut with a dirty sword or plough. An infected wound can cause septicemia and is potentially deadly. This simple question puzzled me because in northern Europe we did not have garlic, myrrh or powerful oregano, and none of the really potent antibiotic herbs spring to mind as being immediately available. Then I heard a story that suggested a possible answer.

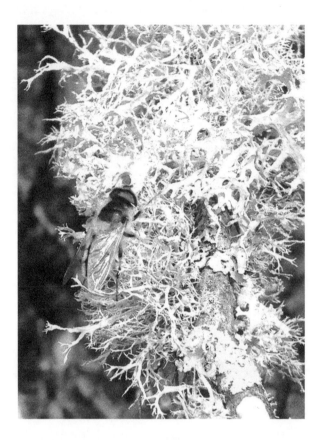

An old wives' tale advises us to smear mouldy cheese onto an open wound. At first, you cannot imagine anything more awful, yet when we remember that the wonder drug penicillin comes from the same family as the mould, which forms the blue veins in Stilton cheese, we can nod at the sage advice.

Now take a look at an old tree and, if the air quality is pure, you will find that the branches are covered in lichen, a primitive symbiotic plant – half algae and half fungus. It is interesting how similar in appearance lichen is to the blue veins in Stilton.

In the olden days, when someone injured themselves, they would sprinkle the wound with dried and powdered lichen, which acted as a natural antibiotic and, indeed, modern studies confirm its significant antibacterial actions. Interestingly, I mentioned this to a friend one day as we passed under an old tree, hanging with lichen in the African bush. He told me that its antibiotic properties are also known in the African tradition. Isn't it fascinating how these plant remedies have been used in exactly the same way by different races, separated by oceans and thousands of miles of land?

Science has caught up with this little treasure trove of protection, and studies show lichen to be very effective against methicillin-resistant *Staphylococcus aureus* (MRSA) with one study concentrating on MRSA in cystic fibrosis patients[1,2] and other bacteria and fungi – including *Bacillus cereus*, *Bacillus subtilis*, *Staphylococcus aureus*, *Streptococcus faecalis*, *Proteus vulgaris*, *Listeria monocytogenes*, *Aeromonas hydrophila*, *Candida albicans* and *Candida glabrata* – were inhibited by lichen plants[3].

It used to be considered excellent against chronic pulmonary conditions such as tuberculosis, and an old recipe suggests boiling the ground lichen in milk with cocoa or chocolate! There are recent scientific studies that confirm lichen's effectiveness against *Mycobacterium tuberculosis*[4]. Another study also demonstrated that lichen and heathers are both effective against the tuberculosis bacteria[5]. Heather, of course, is well known in Scotland as a folk treatment for respiratory and urinary tract infections.

Lichens may also be used as a douche against thrush and more scientific evidence demonstrates that it can treat *Candida albicans* and *Candida glabrata* as well as other infectious fungi such as *Aspergillus niger* and *Aspergillus fumigatus*[6].

Across the world, lichen has formed an important part of the dyeing industry, particularly in Scotland for the famous Harris Tweed. On those islands, the lichen was traditionally fermented in vats of stale urine for about three weeks and used to produce a variety of colours from brown to orange, depending on which species was used.

Sphagnum Moss (*Sphagnum cymbifolium*)

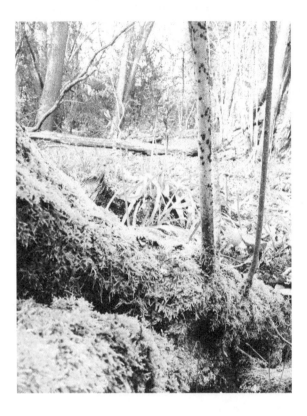

Another insignificant plant which has made an enormous contribution to mankind are the mounds of sphagnum which we find growing abundantly all around us on boggy British soil. The plant structure is made up of tubules, which absorb and hold up to twenty times their dry weight in fluid. Exactly like a sponge, this makes it a very effective dressing for bleeding or suppurating wounds. As usual, nature provides all that we need because the plant is also antibacterial. This is achieved by lowering the pH of the environment which it is in contact with, making it inhospitable to bacteria, which are sensitive to acid.

One study demonstrated sphagnum moss' effectiveness against both gram-negative and gram-positive bacteria such as *E coli* and

Streptococcus spp[7]. This is not breaking news to humanity. Sphagnum moss has been recorded as a wound dressing for at least 1,000 years.

During the First World War, it was collected and picked clean of attached leaves and pine needles, then air-dried and wrapped in muslin before being sterilised by steam. These packs of wound dressings were twice as effective at absorbing blood and pus as cotton wool, and also very soft and comfortable. In the field, these moss-dressing pads were used alongside powerfully antiseptic garlic. The fresh garlic bulbs were sent to the battlefields and pressed out in the field hospitals. The raw juice was diluted in water and added to the dressings before they were applied to battle wounds. This combination was so effective that the wounds suffered no further complications. By the end of the war, Britain was producing up to one million sphagnum wound dressings per month and thousands of lives were saved using these two simple and readily available plants.

The hill women of Nepal used sphagnum moss as pads in the same manner for their monthly periods, and I am sure this is the case around the world wherever this plant grows.

Male Ferns (*Dryopteris filix-mas*)

Medical herbalists do not commonly use the male ferns these days, although the plant has a reputation as an excellent remedy against tapeworms. The root paralyses the worm and, when combined with a strong purgative, the worm is flushed from the bowel. Now this is very interesting: if you look at the tightly curled leaf frond, you will see that it looks exactly like a green worm.

Wild food enthusiasts enjoy the freshly picked and curled fronds when fried with garlic, mushrooms and bacon, or steamed and eaten with butter like asparagus, or even pickled. **However…** one must be careful of this plant as it contains an enzyme which destroys vitamin

B in the body, and other similar ferns are known to cause cancer and blindness when browsed over a three to four month period by animals, so if you do choose to indulge your wild side it would be wise to keep it as a rare treat.

There is a faery myth, which says that if you collect the seeds of this fern at midnight under a full moon on St John's Eve, then you can use these seeds to become invisible and you will also become immensely wealthy. I sniff a faint suggestion of thievery here.

The Oak King and the Holly King

The shifting seasonal balance of light and dark is played out dramatically in the story of the Holly King and the Oak King. The Oak King is the lord of summer, whilst the Holly King rules the winter. The wheel of the year is ever turning with both kings always winning and always losing. The spring equinox being a time of equal hours of light and darkness, is a good place for the story of the battle between the Oak and Holly Kings to begin.

At this time, the strength of the kings is equal but, in the battle between the two, the Oak King wins. During the summer, the Oak is king of the forest, standing tall and proud. His power and strength reach their zenith at the summer solstice, but this is also the day when he falters and the Holly King's strength begins to return. At Lughnasadh, with the first harvesting of the year as the corn is cut, the Holly King has his first victory over the Oak King.

By the time of the autumn equinox, the Oak King has weakened sufficiently that their strength is once again equally matched. The wheel turns towards Samhain, the Oak King dies, his leaves fallen and he stands naked in the forest. The Holly King grows stronger yet. Samhain (Hallowe'en) is the time when folk celebrate and honour those who have died. Holly, the king of darkness, strengthens ever until at the winter solstice he rules in glory with the winter sunlight reflecting off his spear-sharp leaves. He is the only tree bringing colour to the dark woods with his bright red berries. We honour the Holly King by decorating our homes with holly and ivy.

Evergreens like holly were seen as magical plants, appearing to transcend death. While all the deciduous plants have lost their leaves and the land is seemingly dead, the green of the holly reminds us of life. So even as the king of the dark time of year, paradoxically, holly reminds us of life.

Now at the winter solstice, the Oak King is reborn. The sun, at its weakest on this day, grows stronger and to celebrate the strengthening light we decorate our homes with fires, candles and bright or shiny trinkets. Still the wheel of the year turn towards Imbolc, where the light has gathered some strength and the Earth (the Queen) responds by sending up buds and shoots. The Holly King is faltering and the Oak King is gaining in strength, until once again they meet as equals at the spring equinox.

March

The 21st of March marks the spring equinox. At last, after the long winter, the light of the day is of equal length to the darkness of the night. The promises of Imbolc have come to fruition, with renewed life thrusting through the earth. The sap is rising and this is the time of hatchings, bouncing lambs and rabbits, and the soft yellows of primroses and daffodils.

Watching a fox cub concentrating hard on batting a bluebell, one March day, was like witnessing the very essence of springtime innocence and joy. The hedgerow is eagerly waking up to a new year of precious life. This is a time when the natural world is burgeoning with abundant life force.

Cowslip (*Primula veris*)

Around the spring equinox, the cheerful cowslips begin to unfurl their pale yellow flower stalks through the grasses in the meadows. These once abundant flowers were so popular that they are not as easily found on the banks as they once might have been. Perhaps too many were brought into the home with the joy of seeing colour at last after the long dark winters, or perhaps it was the very popular and slightly narcotic cowslip wine that resulted in their population decline.

These days cowslips are protected by law, but in ancient times it is said that the flowers were protected by magical creatures and dedicated to the Norse goddess Freya, the goddess of love, beauty and war. We shall come across goddess Freya again at the other end of the year in connection with mistletoe, but for now I wonder whether the goddess used these flowers as part of her beauty regime; certainly it has been well known by mortal women that an ointment of the flowers and leaves will restore lost beauty and remove wrinkles.

Cowslips are gently sedative and the old herbalists used cowslip flowers to calm 'the phrensies', and even for paralytic ailments, hence its old name palsy wort. When I studied herbal medicine in the 1990s, we were taught that an infusion of the flowers will help the insomniac to drop off to sleep, especially those who were too tired for sleep. They are such dear little flowers that I cannot bear to pick those which I grow in my physic garden. However, if you feel restless or have difficulty sleeping, or even suffer from the headaches of nervous exhaustion, then (if you can bear to pick them) infuse about eight flowers in boiling water and you will have reason to thank them.

Lesser Celandine (*Ranunculus ficaria*)

Lesser celandine is another little joy that welcomes in the springtime. Their dark, glossy green leaves and radiant yellow flowers that glitter in the sunshine brighten up many a dark roadside bank. However it is the roots that interest the herbalist.

There is a long tradition in herbal medicine known as The Doctrine of Signatures. In olden days, people believed that God marked each plant with a sign, indicating how it might benefit humanity. It must be emphasised that medical herbalists no longer refer to The Doctrine of Signatures, and science is entirely disdainful of the idea; however, it is a pleasant pastime to note and compare the structure and habits of a plant with its known healing qualities.

A splendid example is the lesser celandine, which is also known as pilewort. If you pull up a small plant, exposing the roots, you will see that they are almost the spitting image of hemorrhoids (piles)! Indeed, it is for treating this condition that the root is employed. These days we know that the plant is rich in tannins, which tighten and restore tone to flaccid tissues; and so, applied as an ointment, pilewort has been used for centuries to soothe the pain and itching of piles. Another example of The Doctrine of Signatures is the male fern (cf. February), where the curled leaf frond looks just like a curled green worm, the root being used to expel worms.

Cleavers (*Gallium aparine*)

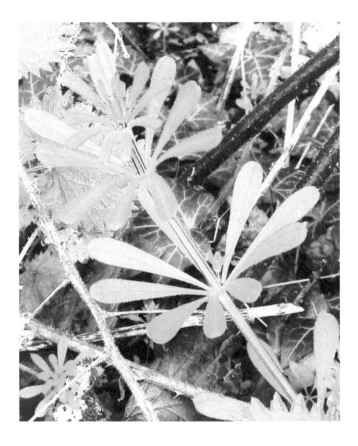

Just starting to grow up every hedge right now is the wonderful cleavers, aka sticky willy or goose-grass. Cleavers is a strong-growing plant, but its structure is weak and thus it needs the woodiness of other hedge plants to support it as it scrambles upwards towards the light.

Modern medical herbalists mostly tend to use this herb as a diuretic, to cleanse the lymphatic fluid and reduce glandular swellings. If for instance a young person comes to see me with tonsillitis, or a woman with premenstrual lumps in her breasts, or even someone with glandular fever, I would consider Gallium to be one of the safest and most reliable herbs to ease these complaints.

It is interesting to bear in mind that the lymphatic nodes filter the debris from the lymphatic fluid, clearing dead bacteria, dead cells and toxins from the blood. The tiny prickles on cleavers remind us of a filter and, as it happens, for centuries housewives would gather cleavers into a ball and use this as a sieve to filter the whey from curds. Gallium is also a notable diuretic, helping to clear the excess and sluggish fluids held in the tissues such as the thighs and hips. The old herbalists used to say that if you wish to remain lean and lank, you should partake of this herb. It is quite delicious, actually.

Eau de Hedgerow

Pull a long strand of cleavers from a hedgerow and roll it into a loose ball, then drop this into a glass of water and leave overnight. In the morning, add a small amount of elderflower cordial. Drink it chilled.

If you persist with this delicious eau, you may well become lean and lank – just like the plant, as it happens.

Nettles (*Urtica dioica*)

When I take people out on herb walks, I love to talk about the ancient enchantment of this land and the associations of magic with plants. People are fascinated, of course, but they don't really buy into these stories until I show them a phenomenon that I call green magic.

There cannot be a hedgerow rover who hasn't been stung by nettles, so of course most people are unenthusiastic when invited to stroke a nettle leaf with their bare hands... However, if you approach the nettles in a friendly manner and pick the leaf quite firmly, once 'captured' it can be stroked like a little pet and it won't sting you. "Ah ha!" some say. "That is because you are only stroking it in one

23

direction." But within minutes everyone in the group is lovingly strok-ing their nettles, up the leaf and down the leaf, topside or underside, along the sides and along the stem. Some even stroke their face and they do not get stung. Green magic! This is a powerful experience that helps people to communicate love and trust to a plant and sub-sequently to fall in love with 'weeds'.

Partly, it is the sting that has made the nettle so valuable in herbal medicine. When the Roman soldiers first invaded Britain 2,000 years ago, they found this island very cold. Apparently, they "seethed nettles in oil and rubbed the herb oil on their bodies to ward off the cold-ness." A good idea. This oil would have dilated the blood vessels and warmed their muscles. Other folk used to flog their arthritic limbs with fresh nettles to cause a flush of circulation. This is known as a rubefacient action.

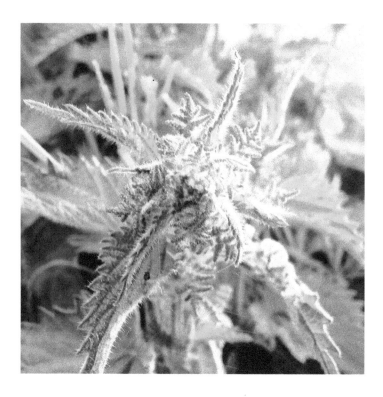

The needles of the nettle inject histamine into the skin, bringing a rush of blood to the site of the flogging. The fresh flow of blood rush washes away accumulated toxins such as uric acid crystals, thus relieving the condition. This type of approach is known as heroic medicine but these days herbalists are a little gentler to our patients. Nettles are also blood cleansers, so we find that a nice cup of nettle tea also washes away the toxic accumulations, but without the pain.

The nettle is a herb, which can be used so safely that it is worth cultivating a little patch in your garden. Why pay for nettle teabags when nothing is better than fresh nettle tea? Simply pick a sprig of nettles, remembering to approach your nettle in a friendly manner or with gloves, and drop it into a cup of boiling water with a few slices of ginger and lemon, and honey to taste. It is the most delicious, invigorating tea.

There are so many recipes that celebrate the nettle. Here in Britain we have all at least heard of nettle soup. Making nettle soup is a wonderful way to celebrate spring, especially when enjoyed with crusty bread and butter.

In Italy, they make nettle ravioli and nettle pesto. The simplest way to eat nettles is to steam the leaves and add a little butter to eat as you would spinach. They taste delicious but have a strangely furry texture, rather like eating tasty green caterpillars. When cooking with nettles only use the young fresh tips, because once they turn to flower they become a bit unpleasant. Nettles were once renowned as a spring tonic. In days gone by, before strawberries were available at Christmas, people would get through the winter largely on preserved meat, stored root vegetables and wrinkled apples. By early spring, those who had survived the winter were desperate for fresh greens and the early wild herbs were eaten as vegetables to cleanse and enrich the blood.

The folk of the olden days would closely observe and emulate nature, and sought to mimic the sap rising vigorously in the trees at springtime. By taking blood-cleansing herbs, they enriched their blood so that their own vigour rose like the sap in the trees, bringing renewed vitality to the person for the busy months ahead.

Nettles are very rich in minerals, especially iron, silica and vitamin K. Vitamin K is essential to help the blood clot, so we see the scientific reason why nettles are used to stop internal bleeding. This is particularly important for women who suffer from very heavy periods. Regular nettle tea will restrict the excessive bleeding as well as replenish the blood with iron, thereby helping to prevent anaemia. We still use nettles for this purpose.

Have you heard of the saying 'hair that grows like weeds'? Alopecia, or hair loss, has several causes but a major one can be iron or silica deficiency. Nettle tops are rich in both minerals so if you want your hair to grow like weeds then make a weedy hair tonic.

In our apothecary, we find nettle to be tremendously successful in restoring hair growth. Stress and a poor diet, both quite common in these speedy times, can lead to falling hair, which for a woman is a disaster. We recommend nettles taken either as a juice or as a tea or tincture. All are successful, but the simplest way is to pick a sprig of nettles, adding another sprig of rosemary and a sprig of horsetail herb; drop these into a cup with some honey and lemon to taste and add boiling water. Drink this three times a day and in time you will be thrilled at your beautiful, abundant and strong hair. Alternatively, make yourself a weedy hair tonic.

Weedy Hair Tonic

Pick a large handful of nettles and boil them in a pot of water for three minutes. When cool, strain the liquid into a jug and add a tablespoon of white wine vinegar. Then pour this mixture over your head every day. Do not wash it out. Your hair should grow thick and strong and the vinegar will make it soft and glossy. Drinking nettle tea daily can further enhance this.

Nettles also have an anti-histaminic effect and we commonly employ nettles every summer to help those suffering from hay fever, usually combining nettles with ribwort (*Plantago lanceolata*) and elder flowers (*Sambucus nigra*). Every part of the nettle plant is useful medically. Medical herbalists use the root to help men showing the symptoms of enlarged prostate glands. Men who use this plant are able significantly to reduce night-time urination and it allows the urine to pass more easily and comfortably; the men whom I have helped with nettle root remain comfortable with their herbal prescription for years, avoiding a rather unpleasant operation.

One of the lesser-known therapeutic parts of the plant is the seed; however, it is commonly used on the continent to increase vitality. For men, it is used to increase the libido and to help strengthen erections, whilst for women the seeds are taken to improve the growth of hair and nails. So we can see this as a seed of love, increasing female beauty and male vitality. The seeds are also taken to support recovery after long illnesses as they are rich in micronutrients and omegas. The dose is three teaspoons taken daily, ideally over porridge oats.

The Horse Dealer

There is a lovely story about an unscrupulous horse dealer who fed an old nag with nettle seeds and oats for a few weeks, whereupon the horse was soon looking glossy and splendid enough to be sold for a bagful of coins. However, once back on a diet of grass, the beautiful horse reverted (as if by black magic) into an old nag, by which time the horse trader had unfortunately moved on.

Now, the story continues... The doctor of an old-age residence heard of this sorry tale and ordered the nurses to add nettle seeds to the residents' porridge, and sure enough they all soon became alert and lusty. The alertness might be on account of the essential fatty acids in the seeds, which are known to enhance brain function. I don't know the pharmacological reason why they became lusty, but that is how the story is told – perhaps it was the extra vitamins and minerals. Another herb said to bring lustiness to older folk is the root of sweet cicely.

Discovery of the Medicinal Properties of Plants

Not only have humans used plants as food and medicine throughout our evolution, but we have always woven together plant medicine and spiritual matters, so that healing was considered a sacred art. To heal is to preserve life and this may still be regarded as a sacred vocation. Plants have been referred to as God-given medicines and, in indigenous cultures, the shaman or Wise One of the tribe is the person in communication with the spirits, or the gods, or the divine. This has always been so.

It is commonly believed that the ancient people discovered the healing properties of each plant through the process of observing animal behaviour, and then adopting a trial and error method. This means that if you were ill, you chewed on a plant and either got better or died, thus knowledge was accumulated. Personally I do not subscribe to that theory, but in truth we shall probably never know. One way to get some idea of what might have happened all those thousands of years ago is to listen to what contemporary indigenous cultures have to say about their plant medical knowledge.

Do bear in mind that herbal medicine is very ancient and, although healing practices were quite different thousands of years ago compared to modern medical herbalism, indigenous shamanic practices have not changed. So that is where we go to find out how the medicinal properties of plants were discovered.

If you look at every indigenous culture the world over, they all have or had a medicine man or woman within the tribe or the village. One of the major roles that this person performed was to go into trance and learn from the spirit of each plant, so that the plants themselves would instruct as to how they should be used to heal the people. Even today, if you ask a Peruvian shaman or a Sangoma from Africa, a Native Indian from America or an Australian Aboriginal healer, how they learned about the powers of the plants, they will consistently tell you that "the plants teach us."

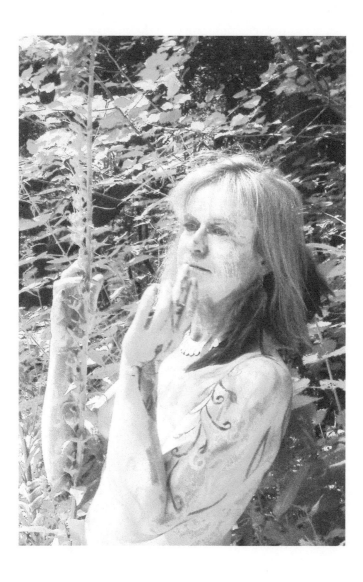

It was very normal for our ancient ancestors to interact with the natural world in a way that we have almost completely forgotten. Whereas we engage our logical and analytical left-brain so effectively, it is understood that older or more indigenous cultures use both left and right cerebral hemispheres, allowing them to view the natural world quite differently to us. Theirs is an animistic worldview. They enjoy much more of a dialogue between the human and the environment. For instance, the San Bushmen of the Kalahari would communicate with the animals before they set out to hunt. In the animistic world view, every river, well, mountain, flower, animal, rock or fire has a spirit with which we can communicate. The world is alive with spirit and intelligence. Everything has meaning.

In my parents' South African home, not a beetle can fly into the house without Constance, their Xhosa housekeeper, interpreting the meaning of that event with fascinating conviction. Constance also has an aunt who is a Xhosa Sangoma, and this lady prescribes herbs by dreaming which herb she is to use for her client: she says that the plant she needs comes to her in her dreams.

In the mainstream Western world, communication with plants has been sniggered at for hundreds of years; but now there is plenty of scientific evidence to support the fact that plants do respond intelligently to our communication. If we lose the willingness to engage with the spirit of nature, we deny ourselves the opportunity to experience the world as so fundamentally enchanting that it can radically change our experience of life from the mundane to the magical.

Beauty, innocence and a vibrant imagination build within us a heavenly inner world of magical enchantment, peace and joy, which can radiate from each of us, spreading to our work, our home life and the way we live our lives. Imagine how the world would change if we all viewed nature through an animistic, sacred and magical lens.

The Wise Ones knew how to communicate with the spirits of the plants, so they learned how to use these plants wisely. This knowledge was passed from shaman to apprentice down countless generations over thousands of years, to the herbalists of the Druids, to the wise woman of medieval times, to the apothecaries of the 17th century, the still rooms of the great houses in the 18th century, to the pioneers of America, the peasants of rural Europe and to the medical herbalists of our time.

One of the ways that we can easily become re-enchanted with the land is through using common hedgerow plants in our daily lives, actually going out to collect them. In this way, we move through the hedgerows with the seasons, connecting to the Earth cycles again with our bodies and minds. We once again tune in to the thrill of the changing energies of the seasons – the nostalgia of autumn, the silence of deep winter, the anticipation and expectation of early spring and the excitement of summer in its fullness.

The harvesting experience is profoundly different if one simply picks herbs, compared to when harvesting with a sense of the sacred. It is one thing to know that you want to collect elder flowers and off you trot to pick a basketful of flowers. It is a completely different experience when you send a message to the elder before you even leave home, telling her that you would like to harvest some of her flowers to use for healing. Once you arrive at your destination, you might approach the tree gently and respectfully, talking quietly to her as you enter into the tree's 'space'. Standing in front of the tree, you might address it in your own way. I speak to the goddess of the elder tree, Helda Moer, thus:

> "Beautiful Goddess Helda Moer, who lives in the elder and protects her. Beautiful tree, of white flowers and black berries, I approach you in deep respect and in joy to gather your bountiful fragrant flowers once again, so that I may use them for the healing of others. I honour your ancientness, your wisdom and your ability to heal the eyes, the nose, the skin and the fevers. Please show me clearly exactly which flowers I may pick and which I should leave alone."

Somehow I am drawn to picking some flowers but feel compelled to leave others alone, and I know when it is time to move on to another tree. Plants will give willingly, but we must ask politely. I have noticed that when a plant has been asked, the leaves, twigs or flowers almost spring off the branches, as compared to when they are not asked and you have to struggle to wrench them off. Of course, we can just take the plant part, but it is not the same as when the plant gives of itself willingly. There is a sense of co-operation between the herbalist and the herb, both in the donating and the healing.

Don't forget to thank the plant earnestly, too, for donating its body parts to you for your healing cabinet. Some people like to leave a gift of, say, tobacco or chocolate. I tend to sing a song or just talk gently to the plant while I am picking her, a bit like talking to a cat whilst combing him. Please bear in mind that one should only take a very small percentage of the flowers or fruit, leaving the vast majority to the birds and insects. Nature is so bountiful that it is quite easy to find enough herbs a little further down the track.

April

The Christian date of Easter is calculated according to the tradition that Jesus was resurrected around the time of the Jewish Passover, which is celebrated on the first full moon following the spring equinox.

According to St Bede (673-735 AD), long before his time the Anglo-Saxon pagans honoured the goddess Eostre in the month of Eosturmonath, which is Paschal month in the ecclesiastical calendar. He writes that Paschal time is known by her name and celebrated as Easter. The Germanic goddess Eostre represents the rebirth aspect of the cycle of the year when life springs out of the earth and from the womb. Thus April has long been celebrated as the time of fertility and new life. Even our female hormone oestragen derives its name from the fertility goddess Eostre. It seems that later the goddess became associated with the fertile hare, who is also associated with the moon. Both the hare and the moon were said to die daily so that they may be reborn, recalling that Easter is very much a lunar and resurrection celebration. Eggs represent a time of potential, the hatching of chicks, of ideas and new beginnings.

Chickweed (*Stellaria media*)

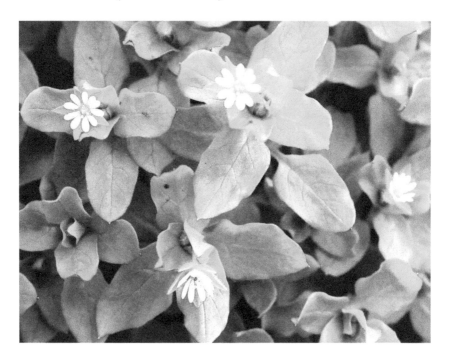

In the garden, chickweed is quite an unloved weed yet highly valued by herbalists who describe it as a 'refrigerant'. You can experience this yourself on a summer's day by placing your hot cheek against a soft mound of chickweed. Immediately you will notice how cool and soothing the plant feels against your skin and this makes it a very comforting herb for hot itchy skin conditions, especially eczema. The herb soothes and cools itchy skin, whilst repairing the damage caused from scratching. It is incredibly safe and we have wonderful results with infant's eczema and nappy rash.

At home you can quite easily pick two large handfuls of the plant and add it to a teapot of boiling water. This infusion may be added to a bath if you are sunburnt or, when cool, sponged over an area that may have been burnt or is suffering from eczema. The infusion can also be drunk hot or cold to soothe inflammation of the digestive tract such as stomach ulcers or gastroenteritis, or you may prefer to snip it into your summer salads.

Chickweed is also very effective as a poultice for infected sores, which have pus deep beneath the skin. In this case you should certainly see a doctor or medical herbalist, but if you happened to be in a position where you were unable to access such expertise then you could take the herb and wrap it in muslin or a clean cotton cloth. Dip the pad into very hot water and allow it to cool such that you can squeeze out the excess water, then apply it to the sore. Leave it until the pad cools then repeat. The poultice should soften the skin and help to draw the pus to the surface so that it bursts.

It would also be a good idea to disinfect the wound with a tincture of myrrh or *Calendula*. If you don't have either to hand, take a leaf out of the book of the front-line hospitals during the First World War: crush a clove of garlic, soak it in half a glass of water and wash the wound with the garlic liquid.

Daisy (*Bellis perennis*)

There is an old saying that, "when you can put your foot on seven daisies, then spring has come." The dear little lawn daisy has long been ignored as a medicine, but its older names bruisewort or poor man's Arnica tell us that it once had a place of importance in its relationship with the common man.

As an aside, you have probably noticed that several herbs have the suffix 'wort' attached to them. So far we have had elfwort, palsywort, pilewort and bruisewort. 'Wort' is simply the Anglo-Saxon word for herb or plant, derived from 'weord' or 'wyrt'; a garden was a 'weord-yard' or a 'wyrt-yard'. People would name plants by description of their properties, so we also have motherwort (a plant helpful in childbirth), St John's wort (the plant that flowers on St John's Day), or lungwort (a plant used in the past for tuberculosis). The name 'daisy' comes from 'day's eye', which refers to the way daisies seem to gaze adoringly at the sun as it moves across the sky during the day. When the sun sets or clouds cover the sun, they close their petals and bow their heads.

Lawn Daisy Footbath or Poultice

This is very useful for treating sprains or bruises. It is as simple as gathering a handful of daisies and dropping them into a teapot of boiling water. After ten minutes, add this tea to a footbath of tepid water and immerse your sprained foot in the water for about twenty minutes.

To make a daisy poultice that can be used for bruises on less convenient body parts, use a saucepan instead and take the hot daisies from the saucepan and place them on a clean piece of muslin, wrapping roughly into a square shape. Now dip the daisy poultice into the daisy infusion, squeeze until it no longer drips and apply it to the bruised area, holding it for several minutes and then re-immersing in the warm water. This should be done several times through the day but you will not fail to be impressed by how quickly the swelling reduces.

This brings us to an environmental point: why would we use very expensive Arnica? This plant grows in the delicate ecosystems of the high Alps and it is an endangered species, so it makes far more sense to use our own little *Bellis perennis*, which thrives abundantly in our own lawns!

Wild Garlic (*Allium ursinum*)

Wild garlic is not a herb that herbalists tend to use in our dispensaries, however it is certainly a plant that we look forward to using in our kitchens. It is very easy to find wild garlic or ransoms: we just look for old undisturbed woodland and then follow our noses. In April, the flowers open and release such a pungent odour of garlic that you can even smell it as you drive past.

Some time ago, I showed a friend a large area of wild garlic. At the time he was suffering from a sinus infection and as soon as I told him that these have very similar actions to cultivated garlic, he picked a few flower heads and ate them at once! His grandson stared at him in amazement and was terribly impressed when my friend's sinuses immediately cleared. His grandson reminded me recently that he had also eaten the wild garlic with his granddad, and it had completely cleared his hay fever sinus congestion; he told me that he had remained free of hay fever for weeks afterwards.

Wild garlic is a respiratory disinfectant and can be used to treat mild chest and sinus infections and coughs. It is also used for dysbiosis, which is an overgrowth of the unfriendly bacteria or yeast in the gut and one of the main causes of bloating, gas and fermentation. The leaves, flowers or bulbs will kill threadworms, and are even more effective in lowering blood pressure and cholesterol than kitchen garlic[8]. When medicating oneself with wild garlic, I think the best method is to 'let food be your medicine, and medicine be your food'. In other words, eat a lot of it. The leaves and flowers are absolutely delicious. I find the flowers add a lovely pungency to salads or sprinkled over new potatoes with olive oil and chopped olives. The leaves can be turned into pesto, or eaten with a chicken and mayonnaise sandwich, or a cheese and tomato sandwich, or crushed with butter and melted into jacket potatoes. Some people like them in a peanut butter sandwich. Delicious recipes abound for this plant, with chefs almost falling over themselves to offer us new and exciting wild recipes. A smooth, green wild garlic and potato soup in a chicken stock, enriched with double cream and eaten with crusty bread is a memorable spring time culinary ritual.

Wild Garlic Pesto

Wash a handful of freshly picked wild garlic leaves and pat them dry.
3 tablespoons of grated Parmesan cheese
3 tablespoons of pine nuts
1 cup of extra virgin olive oil

Roughly chop the wild garlic leaves then add to the blender with the olive oil and pine nuts. Whizz in the blender to the consistency of your choice. Then stir in the Parmesan cheese. This pesto is delicious with grilled or roasted lamb, chicken, salmon or pasta with fresh cherry tomatoes.

Caution: Please make absolutely sure that you are harvesting the correct plant. Wild garlic looks very similar to Lily of the Valley (*Convallaria Majalis*), which affects the heart.

Also, please be aware that the land may belong to someone and it may not be legal to collect plants there. Finally, please harvest with consideration for the plants themselves: only collect a little, so that your enjoyment of the plant does not negatively impact on the survival of the plant population. In the past, shamans and herbalists would always ask a plant's permission to collect its leaves, bark or roots and would leave a gift in exchange. Even if you think that's a bit odd, you can silently thank the plant, which at the very least offers a token of respect towards the living being that is donating some of its body parts for your food or healing.

Garlic Mustard or Jack-by-the-Hedge
(*Alliaria petiolata*)

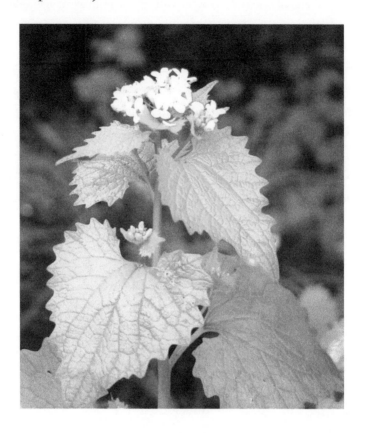

This is a delightful find if you are of the wandering kind who packs a thermos flask and a few sandwiches to sustain a long walk. This very common little plant is generally to be found tucked away under a hedge, looking as inconspicuous as possible, in that way avoiding attention and devouring. But once it is discovered, the wayfarer looks eagerly for Jack-by-the-hedge thereafter. The soft green leaves taste fairly strongly of garlic with enough heat to add 'mustard' to the name. They are delicious with cream cheese on oat biscuits, tossed into a herby omelette, no doubt very nice with sour cream and smoked salmon, laid on a cheese and tomato sandwich or in spring salads.

It is to the sharpness of the flavour and the heat of the leaf that we turn when we consider its medicinal values. In the days of country peasants, they would eat this herb with their salt fish, and it was given the name 'sauce alone'. Culpeper tells us that it aided digestion of the crudities of salt fish and the other corrupt humours of the digestive tract, thus we can consider it a herb that aids digestion. The heat of the herb suggests exactly what Culpeper tells us it is valued for, and that is "to cut and expectorate tough phlegm." The herb was valued in the past to treat sore throats, pneumonia and coughs. Indeed, a chest infection craves garlic, which is powerfully antibiotic and antiviral. So this herb kills the invading bacteria, dislodges the mucus in which the bacteria proliferate, promotes the expectoration of the infected mucus and dilates the bronchi.

For Chest Infection

If we wish to avoid antibiotics, then a really fabulous snack would be a herb sandwich.

Toast some rye bread and rub the toast on both sides with a clove of garlic. Mash an avocado and include in the mash plenty of garlic mustard and wild garlic if you can find some, as well as a quarter teaspoonful of grated, fresh horseradish. Pile the mash onto the toast and eat.

You will immediately feel your bronchi opening and responding gratefully to the herbs (although you may be slightly whiffy). But you will need to persist as the bacteria and viruses won't give up after just one snack.

Before antibiotic medicines were invented, we can only imagine the danger of having open leg ulcers in a society where bacteria were rampant and open sewerage common. The crushed leaves were applied as an antiseptic poultice to open sores to prevent fatal septicaemia. The last official recommendation of this appears to have been in 1838, but it may be that we are returning to the idea a mere two centuries later.

Green Ointment

With bacteria becoming more resistant to antibiotics each year, it may be prudent to extract some of these leaves with bee's wax and olive oil to make a green ointment of antiseptic qualities.

Collect and chop a handful each of garlic mustard and wild garlic. Place in a bain marie (a heated water bath) with any kitchen oil such as sunflower or olive oil, and infuse the herbs into the warm oil for at least two hours. Then press out the oil, reserving the oil and discarding the herbs; this process can be repeated three times so that you have a triple extract of oil.

Once the herbs have been strained from the warm oil, add two teaspoons of beeswax to 80 ml of the oil, and very gently allow it to melt into the oil on top of the cooker.

Now add 20 drops of lavender essential oil to the bottom of a sterilised 100 ml glass jar. Pour the hot oil/wax into the jar and immediately loosely screw on the lid. Once cooled, the lid should be tightly screw on.

Ground Ivy or Ale Hoof (*Glechoma hederacea*)

What a strange name! Long before the days of hops, this plant was used by the Saxons to flavour and clarify their ales, and as such was probably quite a prestigious herb. It lost its prestige during King Henry VIII's rule when hops were introduced, which is a fascinating tale since the people and even Parliament thought hops to be evil or unwholesome, and banned for a time.

The word ale is derived from 'ol' which was a Scandinavian word for a brewed beverage. The Saxons and Celts brewed their ales from ground ivy, wormwood, heather, marjoram and honey; but when hops were introduced to the brew, it became beer, after the German and Dutch 'bier'. The changeover from wholesome herbs to hops was much lamented, as we see John Evelyn saying, "Hops transmuted our wholesome ale into beer, which doubtless much alters its constitution. This one ingredient, by some suspected not unworthily, preserves the drink indeed but repays the pleasure in tormenting diseases and a shorter life."

So, let us return to the wholesome herb then. I think of this plant as English eucalyptus as it is used for similar purposes. Gerard (1545 – 1611) recommended it for the "humming noyse and ringing sound of the eares", or the tinnitus that bothers so many people. He suggests putting the leaves into the ears, but I have to admit that I cannot imagine any London banker wandering around the city with *Glechoma* trailing out of his ears, much as the image amuses me.

I have, however, found it to be very helpful for those who suffer from sinus congestion or blocked ears, and occasionally for tinnitus and temporary deafness. In fact, I once managed to restore someone's sense of smell with this herb – not by trailing it from his nose but given as a tincture. This is probably because the plant dissolves the mucus congestion from the respiratory tract, particularly the upper respiratory tract. One old remedy suggests a certain cure for migraine is to sniff an infusion of ground ivy up the nose. This is said to clear the head and ease a headache, and I am sure an infusion of ground ivy, with elder flowers and some feverfew, would aid sinus headaches.

Gypsies used to boil the herb for twenty minutes, strain it and apply it to infected eyes. I see no reason why this would not make an excellent cure, as the herb is both cooling and antiseptic.

Shepherd's Purse (*Capsella bursa-pastoris*)

This is an insignificant, weedy little thing, which is a blessing to those who use it. Its major value to herbalists is its ability to stop bleeding. It can be used to halt the bleeding of kidneys, lungs, the gut and the uterus. I have found it to be particularly helpful for those who suffer from interstitial cystitis (IC), which is a horrible condition for which there seems little cure, and also with little understanding of its causes.

People who have IC often have ulcerations and chronic inflammation of the bladder with bleeding. Some people also void mucus in their urine, indicating an inflamed and irritated bladder wall. I had a patient who could not endure car journeys because the vibration would cause her great pain and discomfort. With the use of shepherd's purse in her herbal formula, her bladder calmed down and long car journeys were no longer a problem.

With its ability to stop bleeding, particularly in the pelvic region, we value it for those with heavy menstrual bleeding or for those who menstruate for abnormally long periods of time. Of course, the underlying reason does need to be assessed, as in the case of fibroids or other more urgent causes. But in the meantime shepherd's purse is a blessing.

Plants of the cruciferous (cabbage) family will block the thyroid hormones, and we can use this to the benefit of our patients who have a mildly overactive thyroid, but do not want to take mainstream medication. I have found that *Capsella*, belonging to this family, is beneficial for people with this condition, while we try to resolve the rather difficult underlying autoimmune condition.

In the old days, this little weed was fed to caged birds to keep them healthy. Poor little creatures, thank goodness we don't do that anymore; but perhaps you may not weed your garden too vigorously so as to let the wild birds feast.

Celandine (*Chelidonium majus*)

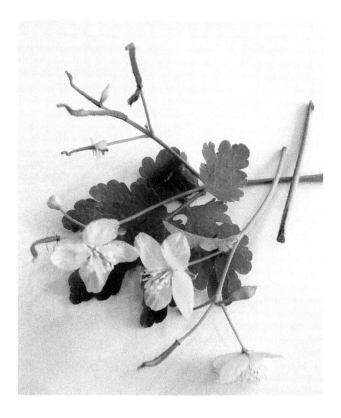

This is not a plant which is often used internally, although it has an excellent reputation for problems related to the liver and gall bladder. Mainly, I have employed this herb to get rid of warts, for which is excellent in doing the job. This very pretty plant belongs to the poppy family and is a delight in a cottage garden. Looking at the plant, you will notice that it has bright yellow flowers and softly scalloped leaves; but it is when you pluck the stem that you find a bright orange sap, which oozes generously. The slender stem and bright orange sap allows you to dab the juice precisely onto the wart, clearly marking where the sap covers the wart. Do this daily and within a few days or a week, depending on its size, the wart will disappear without a trace or any discomfort. The sap may be used in this manner for ringworm and small corns.

The ability of the sap to eat away at excessive tissues was valued by the herbalists of previous centuries for the clearing of cataracts. Culpeper gives his usual scathing scorn of the physician's methods, instead recommending the mixing of the sap with milk and dripping it into the eye to remove the cataracts.

Caution: I strongly urge you not to do this. Our physicians have moved on since 1653 and laser treatment is safe and effective.

The name 'chelidon' is derived from the Greek word for 'swallow', and some believe that this is because the flowers come and go with the swallows. But Culpeper had another idea. He believed that swallows healed the eyes of their young using the herb and he goes on to relate a gruesome experiment: describing how he used a needle to prick out the eyes of young swallows in their nests, he noted that the parents did indeed repair their eyes, he presumed, with this herb.

May

The ancient fire ceremony of Beltane is one of the most joyous festivals of the year. This is the fertility festival, celebrating the union of the god and goddess. At this time of the year, the flowers are showing off their colours, flirting with the bees who fertilise them and then bring an abundance of honey and fruit to the land. The land is drunk on love, and love brings new life.

On the day of Beltane, the village people would go out into the hedgerows to collect May blossom to dress the May Queen. Throughout the day, there was much charging about on horseback and other revelries. When the sun sank below the horizon, upon every hilltop right across the whole island of Britain, people lit the Beltane fires; through these fires they drove their cattle, blessing them and cleansing them of lice and fleas.

The folk would jump over the flames, couples would dance through the flames, pregnant women might step between the fires perhaps asking for an easy birth, and young girls skipped through hoping to meet their future husbands. They danced around the Beltane fires celebrating the union of the god and goddess and the fertility of the land, and later couples would slip off and make love in the fields. The children born of this Beltane night were known as 'merry-begots'. The next morning, a small amount of the cold ash was taken back to family hearths and fields to fertilise the land, bringing the magic home. This is the time of love, fertility and abundance.

Hawthorn (*Crataegus spp*)

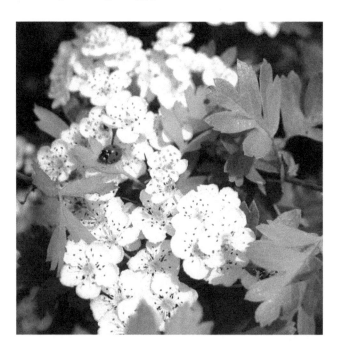

The merry month of May can hardly be mentioned without discussing the hawthorn tree, also known as May blossom. Some people still say that only witches can bring May blossom into the home with impunity. Not very long ago there was a rather unreliable witch test, a saying that if you bring May blossom into the home your mother will die; but if she didn't die, then you were surely a witch! This theme seems to run through many white blossoms such as cows' parsley, with many white flowers having country names such as 'mother-die'.

Looking at the deeper stories and medical uses, this is a tree of the heart. Therapeutically, we know that hawthorn reduces blood pressure by dilating the blood vessels supplying the heart muscle, that way delivering extra nutrients to the cardiac muscle. Hawthorn takes care of the old and tired heart. But hawthorn is so much more than that; it is a tree of the heart of every level.

Let us begin this amazing story by appreciating the generosity of your heart. The cardiac muscle has contracted approximately seventy times every minute of your life and you can quite understand that, after about seventy-five years, the muscle becomes fatigued. With clogging and hardening of the arteries, the heart has a harder job pumping the blood around the body and, because it has to work harder, the muscle enlarges, requiring extra nutrition. By gently dilating the coronary blood vessels, hawthorn allows more oxygenated blood and nutrients to be delivered directly into the cardiac muscle, giving it the necessary strength to continue its work for the last years of life. For similar reasons, herbalists also find this plant helpful for sportsmen or those with weak muscles, as it helps to deliver oxygen to the muscles.

The dilated arteries also reduce blood pressure and relieve the effort required to continue pumping blood around the body. Hawthorn berries and leaves are rich in natural constituents called bioflavonoids, which strengthen and protect the cardiac blood vessel walls themselves, in that way protecting the body against blood clots and stroke. Hawthorn is a very safe herb to use. If you do have high blood pressure, it is perfectly safe to take a little hawthorn brandy each day.

Hawthorn Brandy

To make hawthorn brandy, gather the haws and some leaves in autumn. Place them in a wide neck glass container and just cover with brandy. Place the jar in sunlight and gently shake each day for at least three weeks. Then strain the leaves and berries from the brandy and keep the hawthorn brandy in a dark cool place. It is safe to take half a small wineglassful (approximately 20 ml) daily.

Traditionally, herbalists tend to use the berries and leaves for the physical heart, and the flowers and leaves for the emotional heart. Many are the times when a kindly mother has asked me if I have anything for her teenage daughter who has just experienced her first break-up with a boyfriend... I usually make a formula of herbs with hawthorn flowers, rose petals and vervain (which we say is as comforting as a mother's hug). Here the hawthorn tree is associated with the emotional heart and love.

The Celtic celebration of Beltane falls around the 1st of May, as does the blossoming of hawthorn, hence its common name 'May'. Beltane is a celebration of thanks for the fertility of the land and in older days involved a fertility rite where the 'bride' was dressed in May blossom. In the morning of Beltane eve, the young people of the village would go 'a-Maying' to collect the bowers of May flowers which were to be used as the dress for the May Queen. Whilst they were collecting the blossoms for the festival, there was quite a bit of rustling in the bushes and a new crop of villagers was conceived that day. So we see hawthorn associated with the physical sharing of love.

Hawthorn also represents the spiritual heart and is strongly associated with Glastonbury Abbey and the Christian faith. Jesus brought the message of unconditional love, forgiveness and inclusiveness into our world. He had a wealthy uncle called Joseph of Arimathea who made his money by trading tin from Cornwall and it is said that he knew Glastonbury well. There is a legend saying that after the crucifixion Joseph and a small group fled in his ships from Jerusalem to Britain where they disembarked on the island of Glastonbury (the sea level was higher 2,000 years ago). The exhausted group walked up Wearyall Hill ('weary-all') and requested a miracle of Joseph, to show that this was God's will. He struck his staff into the soil and it miraculously took root, sprouted leaves and grew into the tree that became known as the Holy Thorn. Joseph ended his days in the tiny Christian community that he established at the foot of the Tor, but the Holy Thorn lives on.

A few cuttings of the old tree still survive as very old trees in the Glastonbury Abbey grounds, and they flower both in May and December, as the Mediterranean Crataegus species do. A sprig of the blossom is sent to the Queen's table each Christmas. As an aside, the legend says that Jesus himself came to England with his uncle several times during his 'missing years' and may have taken instruction from the British Druids. During one of his visits to Glastonbury he is said to have built the first Christian church and dedicated it to Mary, his mother; thus, after Israel, Britain is known as the holiest land in Christendom. Glastonbury Abbey stands on the site of that first church and William Blake's much-loved hymn, Jerusalem, honours that legend:

"And did those feet in ancient time, walk upon England's mountains green? And was the holy Lamb of God on England's pleasant pastures seen? And did the Countenance Divine shine forth upon our clouded hills…?"

Also known as whitethorn, or simply thorn, this is one of the three sacred trees of the druids: the oak, ash and thorn. So even magically, hawthorn is the tree of the heart, opening the heart to love. Observe these trees – they are all quite haggard in appearance, with both thorns and beautiful delicate flowers, and they are able to withstand harsh environments. Like real love, which is not all petals and perfume, the tree endures.

An old weather prediction tells us that, "Many haws, many snaws (snows)."

Lady's Mantle (*Alchemilla vulgaris*)

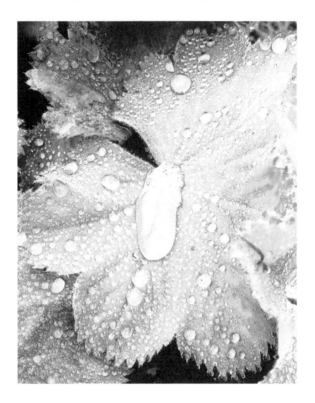

Everyone seems to want to claim lady's mantle as his or her own. The leaves, shaped like inverted umbrellas, collect moisture so that each morning you can find a glistening dewdrop cupped neatly in each one. The plant is named after this dewdrop. It is said that the old alchemists considered dew to be the secret 'prima mater', the first matter of life, hence 'alchemilla'.

However, other writers allude to The Doctrine of Signatures pointing out that the shape of the leaf looks very much like a lady's mantle, or cloak. Like a mantle of protection, it is used specifically to regulate the menstrual cycle and reduce the excessive bleeding that can be so debilitating. On the other hand, Culpeper claimed it as a plant of Venus; but then Christians decided to adopt it as their own, naming it Our Lady's Mantle after the Virgin.

All in all, this pretty little plant has clearly been highly valued for hundreds of years as a medicine. Its specific action is that of astringency where it tightens and heals tissues, making it particularly useful for bleeding or suppurating wounds, diarrhoea, sore throats, but specifically for excessive menstrual bleeding.

Ground Elder (*Aegopodium podograria*)

The English gardener and herbalist, John Gerard (1545 – 1611), rather famously complained bitterly of this plant, being "so fruitful in his increase, that where it hath once taken root, it will hardly be gotten out again, spoiling and getting every yeere more ground, to the annoying of better herbes." And, no doubt, to the annoyance of all gardeners ever since.

This most unloved weed was introduced to Britain as a potherb, possibly by the Romans, and was cultivated by the medieval monks in their physick gardens, where it was became known as bishop's weed or goutweed. Generally, only those who could afford plenty of meat and wine were prone to suffering from gout, and so we must assume that, between the holy fasts, the bishops ate and drank well enough that they suffered from an accumulation of uric acid crystals in their joints, precipitating the necessity to call upon the aid of the weed. Henceforth and even up until 1963, being the last record that I can find of this particular gout remedy, goutwort has been used as a remedy for attacks of gout, rheumatic joints, sciatica and haemorrhoids; however a study in 2012 noted that the essential oil from the flowers had a diuretic effect and instigated uric acid excretion[9].

As a potherb it is actually rather nice, once you get used to its flavour, like nettle, requiring a small expansion of our taste experience.

Ground elder is like a slightly lemony spinach, whereas nettles are more like a richer version of spinach. Since both herbs are excellent for gout, it makes sense to eat them regularly as a vegetable dish if you suffer from the condition. The Italians are familiar with cultivating nettles and the trick for both is to harvest the leaves regularly, so that the shoots remain young and tender.

Ground Elder and Nettle Vegetables

Collect both ground elder and nettle tops. Steam them in a pot with the lid on, in very little water, and add some salt and pepper. When soft, drain them well and add a knob of butter. This dish would go very well with roasted wild Atlantic salmon (with its anti-inflammatory omega 3 oils), followed by a dessert of black cherries, making the entire meal highly commendable for those suffering from an attack of gout. In Switzerland, apparently, ground elder is wilted and eaten with a Gruyere cheese sauce, which sounds delicious.

Ground Elder, Nettle and Wild Garlic Risotto

Gather a handful of each of these weeds, wash and pat them dry. Sautee an onion and add risotto rice to the pan, coating the rice in the oil. Slowly add a good chicken or vegetable stock; stirring the rice absorbs the liquid. When the rice has nearly absorbed all the liquid, add the herbs and allow them to wilt thoroughly. Serve with a sprinkle of dandelion petals and some Parmesan cheese.

If this is more than you can bear, then follow the advice of 20th century monk, Brother Aloysius, by adding a one third cup of the chopped herb to two cups of boiling water, allowing it to steep and drinking a cup twice daily. Other herbalists suggest making a poultice of the herb and applying it directly to the painful part. Culpeper advises that simply carrying the herb about your person is enough to dispel gout.

Should the digging out and eating of the plant not be enough to keep it under control in your garden, why not learn to love those plants that persist? Personally, I find it a very pretty ground cover for difficult areas where not much else will grow, and I allow it to grow under some creamy pink and butter yellow climbing roses where the combination looks every inch the English country garden.

Pellitory-of-the-Wall (*Parietaria officinalis*)

I have tried very hard to grow pellitory-of-the-wall in soil, but it will have none of it. It will only grow in stony places – such as old walls. It is interesting, then, that this herb is best known for its effects against kidney stones. I am not convinced that it would be much help against a large stone, but if you are prone to small kidney stones and gravel, then drinking an infusion of this herb at least three times a day may certainly be helpful in dissolving the stone and preventing it from growing any larger. It is also interesting that the flowers are very discreet and look more like pieces of pink grit that flowers. Its other common name is stone breaker!

Marshmallow (*Althea officinalis*)

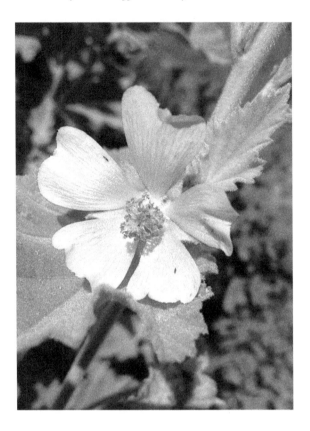

There is something sensuous about marshmallow leaves, so velvety and soft, and this suggests to us the actions of marshmallow. The plant is rich in mucilage, which infuses into water making a slimy and slippery liquid. We refer to this herb as being emollient and demulcent, meaning that it has slimy moisturising and soothing properties. Whilst sliminess may sound a little revolting, it is very soothing to delicate tissues that are raw sore and roughened with inflammation.

This plant can be employed excellently for those suffering from gastric erosions or a stomach ulcer. In this case, the mucus membranes have become eroded and not able to secrete the thick mucus layer that protects the stomach lining from the corrosive action of the gastric acids. In such a state, the stomach wall is vulnerable to being further corroded and a hole or ulcer develops; this can bleed, sometimes with fatal results.

Marshmallow root powder offers a fine and sustainable alternative to the endangered slippery elm bark powder, by becoming thickly gummy and covering the stomach with a lining of plant-based mucilage. In doing so, it protects the stomach wall and allows any ulcer underneath it to heal over again. Combining the marshmallow powder with powder of comfrey leaf will stimulate the healing of the tissues and speed recovery. Of course, it is imperative that the underlying cause of the ulcer be addressed in the meantime.

Those suffering from gastritis or colitis will also appreciate its soothing, slippery actions on the lining of the whole intestine. The herb is equally useful for those who are constipated with dry pellet-like stools. Taking a tea from the leaves or the powdered root in water or milk will help to bulk out the stools, making them slippery and very easy to pass; this is particularly important for those who have haemorrhoids where constipation must be addressed.

Marshmallow is also helpful for people with a dry hacking, rasping cough. By soothing the gastric lining that it comes into direct contact with, demulcent herbs (rather mysteriously) have a reflex action on the lungs and bladder. In doing so, the herb loosens the thick sticky mucus, allowing the dry cough to become more productive and promoting expectoration of the thick sticky mucus which usually harbours pathogenic bacteria. The raw inflamed bronchus is also soothed, so now the vicious cycle of irritable roughness, which promotes the cough and further irritates the tissues to instigate yet another coughing fit, is broken. In this case, I might combine marshmallow root with clove syrup or cherry bark syrup.

This herb also helps those with kidney stones and gravel. These stones scrape and grind their way along the delicate tissues of the urethra, producing excruciating pain, and urine passing over those injured tubes will sting and burn. The mucilage of marshmallow lines the urethra and the slipperiness helps to facilitate the passing of the stone or gravel. Even with cystitis, when the bladder wall is so inflamed and raw that the urine burns painfully, marshmallow soothes and protects those tissues with its slipperiness.

Even further, the powdered root may be used as a drawing poultice when a thorn is embedded in the flesh, or if one has developed a boil, the pus of which needs to be drawn out and expelled. The powder should be mixed with hot water and applied as a poultice under a clean cloth as hot as can be borne by the affected person, and renewed when dried. The heat and drawing action of the herb will pull the pus or the foreign body to the surface where it can be expelled, leaving the flesh clean.

I once met a very organic lady who used to keep a little bowl of fresh marshmallow leaves in her lavatory instead of toilet paper. I thought it rather a nice idea, and it made me think that rose scented geranium leaves might be even nicer.

Marshmallow or its wilder version, mallows, has been valued in the Middle East as a vegetable. They are eaten with eggs and are absolutely delicious. A few young leaves are picked and rinsed, then rolled into a cigar shape, sliced into thin strips and gently fried in butter until wilted; then one adds beaten egg and very gently scramble it all together. The marshmallow leaves taste just like eggs! This is a great way of making eggs go a little further and makes a lovely light evening meal, served with grilled tomatoes that have been seasoned with olive oil and some thyme from your garden.

Infusion for a Dry Cough

5 marshmallow leaves, slightly crushed
½ tsp of dried thyme
I clove
I large spoon of honey

Drop all the ingredients into a teapot with a cup of boiling water and allow them to infuse for twenty minutes, and drink warm.

June

The summer solstice is another fire festival where the bonfires symbolically harmonise with, and give strength to, the sun. It is the longest day of the year when the Sun God is most powerful, but also it is the beginning of his dying as he begins his slow decline towards winter. The Oak King reigns supreme but, as this is the longest day of the year, from now onwards until the winter solstice, imperceptibly at first, his strength begins to wane. For now, there are long warm summer days with an abundance of fruit and food. This is a time of heat, languishing in warm floral meadows and camping out under warm starry skies.

However, we should be aware of what we might stumble upon when wandering about the hedgerows on Midsummer's Eve. It is said that if you sit beneath the elder tree at midnight on Midsummer's

Eve, you may be lucky enough to witness the the Faery Rade. The Rev Robert Kirk describes this procession of the royal faery court thus:

> "The Faery Rade spread out across the sky like a trail of stars, or a fiery comet's tail. Around us the vast expanse of the heavens glowed and glittered, lit by the great round face of midsummer moon. The cold night air rushed by, plucking at my clothing and battering against my face. All around, the people of Faery, in their glorious array, galloped. At times I heard a voice raised in what I took to be song, though such as human voice could never give utterance to. A light was around us, such that I thought the sky must be lit for any mortal who might glance up from the earth below."

Another hedgerow tale advises collecting seeds from the bracken fern under a full moon at midnight on Midsummer's Eve, the seeds of which will make one both invisible and very wealthy. Faeries are often accused of stealing milk and other commodities, so perhaps this is their invisibility trick? Animals made ill through elf magic could be cured with a handful of St John's Wort if it were plucked at midnight on St John's Eve (the Christian Midsummer's Eve).

It seems that midnight on the summer solstice was a very busy time in the hedgerows. One can imagine all sorts of rustling through the bushes, collections of spell craft herbal ingredients, and magical meetings going on. The hedgerow during Midsummer's Eve must have been lively place indeed to spend the night.

St John's Wort (*Hypericum perfoliatum*)

When you look at the flowers of St John's wort, you see an image of the sun with its rays radiating out of its cheerful little floral face. This plant brings light into our lives, both in the modern idea as an antidepressant and anti-anxiety herb, taking away the darkness of nervousness and sadness, but also in the ancient context where it was used to protect again dark and evil forces.

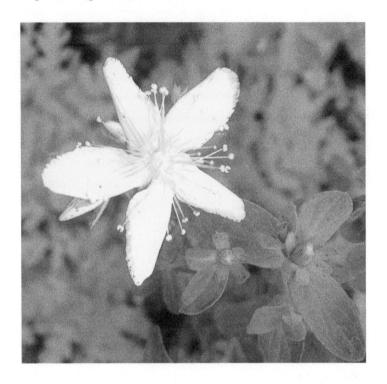

The name *Hypericum* comes from the Latin 'hyper' meaning above and 'icon' meaning spirit. Bunches of the herb were hung over doorways to keep away witches, evil spirits, or it was burned like incense to sanctify an area. When I was a student, we were taught to think of the plant as a restorative to the exhausted nervous system rather than simply an antidepressant. When a person is consumed with anxieties to which they cannot find a solution, their distress turns inward, becoming hopelessness and despair. Here, St John's wort brings relief in the form of relaxing the person while at the same time nourishing and restoring the stripped out nervous system, giving the necessary support to face problems and find resolution or acceptance. Sometimes acceptance is the only option, but finding acceptance can in itself bring peace and healing, which in turn opens the way for new and unexpected opportunities.

Examining the petals and the leaves, we notice that they have tiny dots, which are glandular oil ducts. When the herb is steeped in a base oil such as olive oil for several weeks, the oils leach into the base oil turning it blood red. St John's wort oil has been valued by both modern and ancient herbalists for skin conditions such as burns, sunburn, gastritis or hot inflammatory skin conditions such as eczema. Notice how the hot-red coloured oil is used to treat hot, red conditions.

Gerard recommended this plant for deep wounds and homeopaths today, using the law of 'like treating like', use it for the treatment of puncture wounds; this refers to the perforations in the leaf which suggest (Doctrine of Signatures again) that it would be helpful for puncture wounds. This homeopathic application agrees with the centuries old herbal tradition of using it to treat deep injury by nails or thorns. Today, we tend to suffer less from wounds and more from nervous debility, but the herb and the oil of the herb are very helpful in healing surgical wounds and scars.

Its healing of the nerves is not confined only to the mental nervous system but also our physical nerves. With its antiviral properties, St John's wort makes an excellent choice for post-herpetic neuralgia, or the pain caused by shingles. The antiviral properties are such that the plant is being investigated for its uses in HIV and AIDS[10,11].

Different countries can use herbs for different purposes, and in Germany St John's wort is more valued as a liver tonic than a nerve tonic. Almost all herbs used to treat the liver tend to be yellow in colour. As suggested by The Doctrine of Signatures, the yellow of the plant reflects the yellow of bile. In this case, the plant is used to stimulate the flow of bile in an over-congested liver, thus flushing the bile sludge into the bowel for elimination. It has often been found that a sluggish liver leads to a certain type of sluggishness of spirit and, during the early 20th century, German immigrants used the herb as a digestive tonic to treat melancholy.

Dog Rose (*Rosa canina*)

In June, the bees drone gently amongst the pink and white dog roses, which drape themselves so decorously through our hedgerows. It is one of those hypnotic sounds of a country summer's day.

Herbalists use the petals of roses as a cooling astringent agent. Astringents tighten inflamed watery tissues such as hot, itchy eyes, and diarrhoea, which Culpeper describes so clearly as "slippery bowels"! In these cases, you would add a large handful of petals to a cup of boiling water. Allow it to cool and drink as a tea, or strain through a clean cloth and use as eyewash for conjunctivitis or during the hay fever season. If you have a stomach bug and runny tummy, you can add ½ tsp of cinnamon powder and another handful of bramble leaves to your rose petal tea, drinking three or four cups daily.

The petals are known to calm and cool both the cellular tissues as well as the senses. This is particularly helpful for menopausal ladies who feel hot and bothered. More than just a little bothered, during the menopause women can suddenly experience feelings of great anxiety and depression for no particular reason. Rose petals comfort the emotional heart at these times.

Rose hips are tremendously high in antioxidant vitamin C, and I do wonder why people bother to buy expensive laboratory produced vitamin C tablets when we could follow our grandmothers' example and collect the hips to make delicious rose hip syrup or jam. One cup of rose hip pulp contains more vitamin C than forty oranges! Of course, nature is as clever as ever, offering us rosehips in late summer and giving us just enough time to make and use our own medicines before the cold and `flu season strikes as soon as children return to school.

Consider that in late summer the generous hedgerows provide rose hips and blackberries, both rich in vitamin C, and elderberries, also rich in vitamin C and with powerful antiviral action. It would be very easy to create a delicious and effective immune tonic that would keep our families out of the doctors' surgeries and off antibiotics, probably for the entire winter. In this way we strengthen our immune systems and bodies, rather than weaken them with antibiotics, and emerge stronger after a long winter.

Honey of Rose Petals and Bramble Leaves

Collect a handful of wild, unsprayed rose petals and a handful of bramble leaves, crushed with a pestle and mortar. Place these in a bain marie and gently warm some raw honey. When the honey is soft and runny, pour it over the petals and leaves, leaving it to warm for an hour and allowing it to cool overnight. Then gently reheat the mixture and strain it into a sterilised jar.

Take a teaspoon of this medicated honey frequently whenever you have a sore throat, or apply it to leg ulcers that will not heal.

Rose Vinegar

Collect fragrant rose petals and immerse them in apple cider vinegar for two to three days, until the petals become clear; then press them out, retaining the vinegar, and immerse more petals in the vinegar. After several extractions, the vinegar will have a beautiful rosy fragrance. This can be used in salad dressings or as a cosmetic (see below).

Skin Cleansing Tonic

Dilute 10 ml of rose vinegar into 60 ml of spring water or, even better, rose water. Combine 70 ml of the rose water/vinegar solution with 10 ml of vegetable glycerine and 20 ml of almond oil.

Put all the ingredients into a bottle and shake it vigorously before wiping the liquid over the face with a cotton wool ball as a cooling, cleansing skin tonic. Make small quantities of this tonic so that the water does not go off.

Rosehip and Apple Jelly

500 g of rosehips
1 kg of windfall crab apples
Jam or preserving sugar

Cut up the apples and put them into a pan with enough water to cover, plus two extra cups of water. Cook to a pulp. Place your rosehips into a blender and chop roughly, then add to the apple pulp and simmer for ten minutes; remove the mixture from the heat and leave it to draw for ten minutes before straining it through a jelly bag. This step is very important and you need to strain out all the hairs found inside the rose hips as they can irritate the throat.

Once strained, measure the liquid and allow 400 g of preserving sugar for each 550 ml of juice. Place both in a pan and boil for three minutes. Test for setting on a cold plate and then pour the jelly into warm, sterilised jars.

Rose Petal Sandwiches

In a glass bowl, place a layer of highly scented rose petals on the bottom, then some fresh butter, then overlay the butter with more highly scented rose petals; leave them overnight. In a glass jar, layer caster sugar with more highly scented rose petals and again leave this overnight to absorb the perfume. In the morning, slice white bread thinly, remove the crusts and spread with the rose-scented butter. Now place several rose petals carefully, so that they peep out from the slices. Sprinkle with a little of the rose-scented caster sugar and double over like a normal sandwich.

Serve these with rose-scented tea. These sweet sandwiches are said to have been served at Balmoral tea parties.

The Elder Tree (*Sambucus nigra*)

The beautiful elder tree is one of the most useful plants in the herbalist's materia medica. At this time of year, the tree is heavy with frothy, creamy flower heads, which can be turned into delicious elderflower cordial or champagne, ice cream or fritters. I think of the flowers as one of the quintessential tastes of an English summer.

Elder flowers have anti-inflammatory actions on the mucus membranes of the eyes, sinuses and nasal passages. Again we revisit the old Doctrine of Signatures, now relating to the timing of herbs and ailments. At exactly the same time of year when pollen allergies are ruining summer for so many, the elder flowers soothe symptoms of hay fever such as sinusitis or itchy eyes. It is quite simple to make a tea from the flowers and you can drink as much of this lovely tea as you please to relieve a stuffy nose, making sure to inhale the steam as you do so.

I once attended a workshop in the countryside and was suddenly attacked by terribly sneezy hay fever, with my nose was streaming so much that I could barely concentrate. Luckily there were elderflowers just outside, so I managed to get hold of a cup of boiling water and submerged a flower head of elderflowers in the water. Within twenty minutes of drinking the infusion the symptoms had gone, and when they restarted two hours later I repeated the remedy, and again it halted that hay fever. If you suffer from sore, itchy eyes, then chill the infusion and dip cotton wool pads into the infusion, lie down and gently place the pads over your closed eyelids.

The berries are produced at the end of August, just before the cold and `flu season. These berries are very rich in vitamin C and have strong antiviral actions. For hundreds and probably thousands of years, elderberries have been used against the influenza viruses, and now scientific studies are proving that elderberries boost our immune system[12,13].

It is interesting to compare loosely a study conducted during the 2010-11 influenza season in Russia that showed Tamiflu (Oseltamivir) to reduce the duration of the illness by two or three days[14] with a Norwegian study of the 1999-2000 influenza season where elderberry syrup relieved `flu symptoms four days earlier than the placebo group[13]. Whilst this is not a direct comparison, with a different sample group and different strain of the influenza virus, it does show that the elderberry may be considered a viable option as an antiviral agent to reduce the duration of `flu. The very delicious Elderberry Rob is a cold and `flu remedy, so old that it was considered ancient when the herbals were written hundreds of years ago. Imagine that! A remedy of untold age that is just as effective now against viruses as it must have been all those centuries ago. By comparison, it took bacteria less than five years to start showing resistance to penicillin.

Returning to The Doctrine of Signatures, isn't it fascinating that the anti-inflammatory flowers blossom at the height of the hay fever season, and the antiviral immune boosting berries are available in abundance during autumn, just in time for the cold and `flu season?

The elder tree is strongly associated with magical folk stories. A German tradition tells us that the goddess of weather, spinning and witches, Frau Holle or Hylde-Moer (Elder Mother), lives in and guards the elder tree. If folk wanted to use the wood of the elder, they knew to ask Frau Holle's permission or risk her wrath. The old stories tell us of babies being stolen from the cribs made from elder wood if the father had not taken the precaution of asking permission before cutting the tree. It is said that some babies either failed to thrive, or were switched with faery babies, and although the changelings looked similar to the stolen baby they could be recognised by their evil tempers.

So strong was the belief in the power of this tree, or the goddess who protected it, that in some rural parts of Europe people would doff their caps and greet the tree in passing. I have even read accounts of farm workers refusing to cut an elder tree, so much was their fear of the goddess who lived in that tree. Even today, some people refuse to burn the wood. You see in this example, people not just treating a tree like a tree but as a being worthy of the greatest respect, at least equal with humans. This is very rare nowadays.

Our world is so far removed from these ancient customs that we cannot imagine such notions, but herbal medicine has a very long history, richly entangled with the folklore of times extending far beyond even the Druids. For thousands of years people conducted their lives in accordance with a magical, animistic worldview.

Animism is a belief that all natural things have a spirit and consciousness, and perhaps we scoff at these primitive ideas until we start to take notice of odd events. When I opened Botanica Medica in St Margaret's, we put up a large wooden sign featuring a picture of the elderflowers on one of the outside walls that led down a scruffy alley. Within just a few months, an elder tree had self-seeded itself, directly beneath that picture, and soon the scruffy alley had filled itself with medical herbs — none of which I ever planted. They just moved in. It is said to be very auspicious if an elder tree self-seeds itself in your garden; but when she planted herself right under her 'portrait' we were absolutely thrilled. We call our elder The Goddess Tree and look after her very carefully!

Note that the elder is both black and white: black fruits in late summer and white flowers in early summer. The ancients saw this as a tree of beginnings and endings. At the dark times in our lives when we lose hope, the elder grandmother, also called the Cailleach, can support us through those dark times with her wisdom; and by remembering the soft white flowers of early summer we know that nothing stays the same and there will be lighter times ahead. The wheel is always turning – life, death, life, new beginnings, death of the old, changing, turning, spinning. The elder grandmother teaches us to accept that the wheel of life is always turning. In the death of a situation, we can ask our deepest selves what we would love to be born out of this experience and, by focusing on that, it often manifests.

On a more practical note, the berries have been used by the Scots to dye their tweeds blue, the flowers being used for yellow dyes. The leaves are said to have a peculiar smell, some say like mice nests, but I wouldn't know since I've never sniffed a mouse's nest. Nonetheless, the odour seems to be particularly repulsive to flies, and olden farmers would hang a handful of crushed leaves on their horses' headgear or plant the tree near to barns to ward off flies. Perhaps if flies plague you during your summer barbeque, you might try placing a handful of lightly crushed leaves on the table. Just don't forget to ask Frau Holle.

Elderberry Cordial

Collect ripe black elderberries and, using a fork, strip them from the twigs. Drop a cup of these elderberries into two cups of boiling water and boil lightly. Then use a potato masher to crush the berries, releasing the juices. Add some cinnamon, fresh ginger and cloves, and cover the pot, leaving it overnight to infuse.

The next morning, strain the extracted herbs from the liquid, reserving the liquid. Re-heat this and dissolve as much sugar as will be absorbed by the warm liquid, making a thick cordial. Pour this into a sterilised bottle and, in the winter, take 15 ml in a cup of hot water everyday as an antiviral, protective hot toddy.

Elderflower Fritters

Pick a few elderflower heads. Whisk together a little self-raising flour, an egg and milk to make a light batter. Dip the flower heads into the batter and fry them in sunflower oil until golden, then drain them on kitchen paper. Sprinkle with cinnamon sugar and serve with vanilla or orange ice cream.

Ribwort (*Plantago lanceolata*) and Plantain (*Plantago major*)

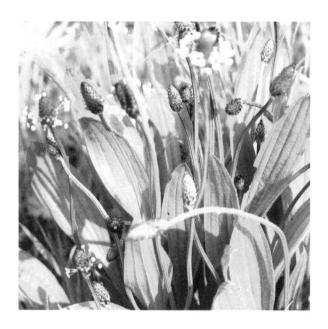

Besides elderflowers, two other plants that we find helpful for hay fever are the very common herbs ribwort and plantain. These plants can be found almost anywhere, in fact they are so common that they became known as 'white man's footprint' by the indigenous people of the countries colonised by the English, because these plants would spring up wherever the white man walked.

Ribwort and plantain can be used interchangeably and they represent another of the refrigerant herbs, which both cool and heal. The leaves cool and soothe the mucus membranes as well as hot skin conditions. The old herbals tell us that this leaf is also good against the bite of a mad dog, but we use it for insect bites or stings, especially nettle stings. Simply crush and rub a leaf over the sting so that the juice covers the sting, or chew it and apply the pulp as a poultice. You will notice the pain receding immediately.

If you are out in the countryside and are suddenly attacked with hay fever, your eyes and nose streaming, look for a ribwort plant (they can be found almost anywhere). Thoroughly chew a leaf and eventually spit out the hard ribs. Within ten minutes you will feel much relieved. It is not delicious, but it does offer a quick and natural antihistaminic effect.

Quick Hay Fever Tea

Take a florescence of elder flowers, four to six crushed plantain or ribwort leaves and a sprig of nettle leaves, adding honey and lemon if you wish. Pop these into a teapot and cover them with a cup of boiling water. When cool enough, drink this tea to soothe your symptoms.

We use plantago juice or tincture in winter too, when people have rough hacking coughs, or thick sticky mucus, which is difficult to expectorate. Plantain soothes the irritated mucosa of the bronchi and the throat, and makes the mucus thinner, so that it is more easily expectorated.

Caution: be very certain before eating wild plants that you are eating the correct plant, and also be aware of areas where dogs might have lifted their legs!

White Willow (*Salix alba*)

For centuries, country folk have used white willow bark when joint stiffness and pains are aggravated by wet and cold weather. Remember how granny would rub her knees and tell us that she could feel the rain coming? "I can feel it in my bones." A cup of white willow tea would have helped her to feel a little more comfortable. As a medical herbalist, I might have added a little ginger to her herbal prescription, which brings heat into the body; you could think of ginger as driving the cold and damp out of the body, whilst the willow brings suppleness. Ginger also has a rich source of natural anti-inflammatory constituents called zingiberol.

A woman once told me that each time she prunes the willow tree her old arthritic dog rushes forward and gnaws on the sticks. For several days he walks around much more easily. Now she never throws the sticks away but keeps them for her dog to chew on whenever he wants to.

In 1899, the pharmaceutical company Bayer was selling a miracle drug called aspirin, which wonderfully killed the pains of headaches and arthritis. Aspirin is derived from the bark of the willow and is rich in salicylates, but the side effects are that it can severely ulcerate the stomach. Now, another herb rich in anti-inflammatory salicylates is meadowsweet but, amazingly, medical herbalists use meadowsweet to heal gastric ulcers. So how, you may ask, can a herb rich in salicylates cure the same ulcers that are caused by aspirin? The reason is that nature provides botanical constituents that protect and heal the gastric membranes in much greater quantities than the salicylates. In this way, the lining of the gut is protected and even healed whilst the salicylates do the job of reducing the inflammation and fever.

Pharmaceutical companies, on the other hand, discovered the anti-inflammatory properties of salicylates, synthesised the chemical and then concentrated huge quantities of it into a single pill, so that the dose is vastly higher than you would find in the whole plant extract; but it lacks the synergistic properties of the other protective constituents. The effects of aspirin are spectacular: the pain disappears within minutes and certainly to a greater degree than if one had taken a tincture of meadowsweet or white willow, but the side effects of aspirin are severe.

Observing the beautiful, soft and gentle willow standing on the river bank with her tendrils flowing with the river tide, our attention drifts towards the ancient Celtic ogham understanding of the tree. Psychically she brings us to our inner river of dreams and we flow back to the source of our inspirations. She helps us to go with the flow of what is, surrendering to the greater flow of life, releasing buried emotions and washing away sadness by helping us to surrender, to let go and flow onwards.

Meadowsweet (*Filipendula ulmaria*)

Just like willow, meadowsweet also loves damp places and I have discovered that it will often grow in hidden ditches. If you are cheerfully wandering along the meadows and you notice a cluster of meadowsweet, take heed for they often warn of an overgrown ditch that you might fall into. But if you do happen to fall into the ditch and badly sprain your ankle, at least the very herb you need will be right there for it is wonderful at easing pains brought on by arthritis or joint injuries. In this case, while you are down, pick a good handful of the flowers and leaves. Once you have hobbled home, make a strong infusion of the herb and when it is cool enough immerse your foot into the herbal waters to reduce the inflammation. If available, also include a handful of lawn daisies for the bruising. You can even drink a cup of the tea whilst you relax and enjoy your footbath.

Meadowsweet is a beautiful and elegant plant, standing with tall, frothy creamy flower heads in the meadows. Her old name Queen of the Meadows honours her beauty, but is also appropriate because queens in the past have loved it as a strewing herb. The cut plant was strewn over the palace floors to release a beautiful marzipan-like fragrance when walked upon, thereby perfuming the queen's chambers and disguising other more unpleasant odours.

Its original name, probably medwort or meadwort, tells us how this plants was used to flavour the delicious honey wine called mead in Britain. Many old herbals sings its praises for "it maketh the heart merry and joyful and delighteth the senses", certainly as a strewing herb at least.

The leaves and flowers are mildly astringent and anti-inflammatory, so they are particularly helpful for diarrhoea when the gut is inflamed as in gastritis, often caused by a gastric infection or by aspirin. In this case it would be very good when drunk as a tea at least four times a day with some chamomile and marshmallow.

The herb is also valued as a diuretic and, when drunk as a hot infusion, will promote perspiration; thus we can use this plant gently to cleanse the tissues through the kidneys and the skin in a similar way to elder flowers. When combined with elder flowers, yarrow and peppermint, this would make a cooling and refreshing tea for those who have a burning temperature or fever.

Caution: Do not use white willow or meadowsweet if you are allergic to aspirin.

Mugwort (*Artemisia vulgaris*)

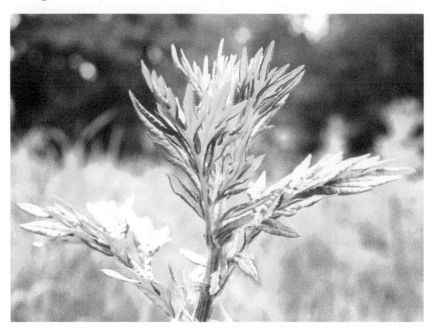

This is another herb with ancient magical associations, and for a very common weed it somehow seems to have collected a lot of stories, surrounding it with an air of mystery and power. The ancients believed that it protected against fatigue, venoms, contagions, wild beasts and evil spirits...

The Lacnunga manuscript, one of our oldest surviving remedy books, is a compilation of Anglo-Saxon medical charms, spells and prayers dating from the early 11th century and recording The Nine Herbs Charm. It addresses mugwort thus:

> "Remember, mugwort, what you made known, what you arranged at the Great Proclamation. Una, you were called, oldest of all the herbs, you prevail against three and against thirty, you prevail against poison and against contagion, you prevail against the loathsome foe roving through the land..."

The authors of the Lacnunga clearly valued this herb for its protective properties against venoms and contagions. The Anglo-Saxons seem to have been very concerned about 'flying venoms', which were blown in on the wind, landing on an unfortunate person and causing disease. The venoms were blown away again by the healer's (magician's) use of song, salt, water and specific herbs such as mugwort.

Today there are scientific studies confirming very powerful actions against bacteria such as *Staphylococcus aureus* and *E coli*[15], malaria[16] and cancer[17,18]. The plant is rich in thujone and 1.8 cineole, two natural plant chemicals known to be powerfully antimicrobial. The plant is also rich in artemisinin, which is valued as an antimalarial agent and may be effective against several types of cancer cells. So although 1,000 years ago the "loathsome foe roving through the land" may well have been plague, we find this amazing weed is also effective against our more contemporary loathsome foes.

Mugwort is famous as a magical herb in these modern days too, as it is said to promote lucid dreaming, the ability to be conscious of one's dreams while experiencing them. According to Carl Jung, our subconscious landscape is revealed to us during our dreams, but most people immediately forget their dreams upon waking so the insight is lost. Drinking mugwort tea seems to allow us to experience and remember our dreams more clearly. Dreaming has been used as a healing therapy since at least the time of the ancient Greeks, and we shall explore this in greater depth when we discuss poppies.

Mugwort Dream Tea

1 part dried valerian
1 part fresh or dried catnip
4 parts fresh or dried mugwort

Take one heaped teaspoon of the mixture and add it to a cup of boiling water. When cool enough to drink, strain and drink this tea thoughtfully, with a prayer or the intention that your dreams will reveal to you what you need to know. You may also like to place a generous sprig of mugwort in your pillowslip to enhance the effect. Wrapped into a cigar-like shape and dried, mugwort also makes a wonderful smudge stick or incense that can promote a slightly altered state for meditation or magical journey work. Some use it to smoke a room where they want to clear the air of any 'bad vibrations'.

Artemisia vulgaris is named after the Greek goddess Artemis, goddess of the moon and of hunting, and this gives a clue to our modern use of this herb. In herbal medicine, it is used primarily as a woman's herb, stimulating the sluggish uterine blood flow that so often causes period pains. Women with congestive dysmenorrhoea (sluggish blood flow) often feel very irritable, bloated and tearful or depressed before their periods. By stimulating the pelvic circulation and improving the liver's ability to clear the build-up of hormones, the blood flow is fresher and the woman feels great relief.

As a bitter tonic, the herb encourages the flow of gastric enzymes and in doing so improves digestion. We find it very helpful for patients with the sensation of fermentation in their guts such as lots of gurgling and smelly gas. By increasing the digestive enzyme secretions, killing unfriendly bacterial overgrowth, encouraging bile flow and thus liver detoxification, the lower digestive tracts is cleansed, leaving the person feeling flatter and much more comfortable in their bodies.

Hedge Medicine and Witches

The common association of hedgerow plants and magic seems to be linked to witches and their cauldrons. Even in my modern herbal apothecary, my patients frequently refer to their herbal prescriptions as their 'brew, potion or concoction'. I have long lost count of the times I have been asked if I am a white witch, to which I usually smile and say that, if anything, I am perhaps a green witch.

Not long ago, people went to great lengths to keep witchcraft away by tying rowan twigs above their doorways, planting elder trees at the four quarters of their gardens or carrying St John's wort or garlic about their persons. Witches and Wise Women have recently become interchangeable, but a few hundred years ago many witches were considered to be sorcerers of the dark arts, and almost everyone used spells to avert black magic.

The Wise Woman, or Cunning Woman, was the village herbalist (and psychologist) who almost certainly also included prayers, incantations and rituals of intention (spells) to achieve her goals. It is quite likely that she sold spells too, with the accompanying words, directions and plant matter. The Wise Woman was the person that the village people went to for healing. Few folk could afford a doctor and often their medicine was as dangerous as the disease. But the people who lived close to the earth trusted the woman who was one of their own, using plants familiar to them.

According to Dr Brian Bates (The Way of Wyrd, Hay House 2004), the male sorcerers or Druids of the British Isles had largely been replaced by priests and monks by 1,000 AD. But women, who were seen as weak and insignificant by the patriarchy in those days, continued their magical practices unnoticed for hundreds of years longer until the Church initiated the infamous witch trials. The herbs healed, but the Church declared that illness was a punishment from God and only God could heal; therefore anyone who gave healing would have been in collusion with the Devil. Thousands of innocent women were either tortured, hanged or burned as witches, sometimes for as small a crime as delivering a baby safely or relieving someone of their pain.

Many herbalists still suffer from a sense of 'inherited trauma', and tend to be a little quiet about their work; even I don't like having to explain to strangers why I am collecting a basket of herbs in the hedgerows. Nevertheless, the knowledge was whispered from mother to daughter, and today we learn it from books and are free to practise herbal medicine. The UK is almost unique in that herbal medicine is legal, thanks to a law passed by King Henry VIII who had great respect for herbal medicine.

The Lacnunga manuscript is a book of remedies about 1,000 years old and within its pages are many prayers to the plants, to charm away illnesses. This may relate to what we now call the power of intention. Indeed, Dr Emoto has shown (The Hidden Messages in Water, Atria Books 2005) that positive words actually change the structure of water into beautiful crystalline shapes, whereas harsh words give the same water a discordant and ugly structure. Since we are 70% water, it doesn't seem so crazy to whisper a powerful prayer or a good intention into a herbal medicine.

However, the Lacnunga teaches us more because the spells address the herbs as beings of power and with great respect. A new science called plant neurobiology is studying plant intelligence and the ways in which plants compute[19]. This young science perhaps represents a return to the consciousness of offering plants the respect they are due. After all, isn't it absolutely magical that we can pluck a weed from the earth, steep it in boiling water and drink it, and become healed of our illness where modern drugs had failed? Plants are beings of power to be respected.

July

Hedgerow flowers are in full bloom now and the nectar is flowing freely. Our lovely bees are using their alchemical skills to turn the nectar into that golden ambrosial liquid that we call honey, so beloved by civilisations around the world that it is almost universally considered to be sacred and magical. Since time immemorial, honey has been the symbol of the sweetness of life and, as such, made into celebratory foods, intoxicating drinks and love potions.

It has wonderful medical virtues too, used to as a natural antibiotic, to stimulate wound healing, suppress coughs and to reduce pollen allergies. Herbalists have for centuries used honey as a medium for delivering herbs: sometimes we mix it with an herb-infused vinegar to create an oxy-mel ('oxy' meaning sharp or acid, and 'mel' derived from Apis melifera, the honey bee).

Honeysuckle, Woodbine *(Lonicera pericymenum)*

Culpeper gets himself into quite a froth over this plant. He starts off by refusing to describe it, as "everyone that hath eyes knows it, and he that hath none, cannot read a description…" Then he launches into a rant, stating that "Doctor Tradition, that grand introducer of errors, that hater of truth, lover of folly and mortal foe to Doctor Reason, hath taught the common people to use the leaves or flowers of this plant in mouth-water [as a mouth wash], and by long continuance of time, hath so grounded it in the brains of the vulgar, that you cannot beat it out with a beetle… Again, if you please, we will leave Doctor Reason for a while, and come to Doctor Experience, a learned gentleman… take a leaf and chew it in your mouth, and you will quickly find it likelier to cause a sore mouth and throat than cure it."

In Sussex a gentleman was considered lucky to possess a honeysuckle stick, especially when courting the lady of his choice. The stick was actually a hazel staff around which a honeysuckle had entwined itself. Once the honeysuckle, or woodbine, was removed, the hazel rod had a twisted appearance, and this magically predisposed the lady to fall in love with him, no doubt to become intertwined with him by sympathetic magic.

Other country traditions are emphatic that honeysuckle should never be brought into the home, for a wide variety of reasons including that it will give young girls erotic dreams, it is unlucky for the family, it will prevent a second crop of hay or that it can give everyone a sore throat simply by being in the house. Despite all these various traditions we continue to love honeysuckle, probably because of its sweet nostalgic fragrance reminding us of romantic garden bowers. The Elizabethans saw it as a symbol of sweet love, where the lovers were entwined in each other's arms, enveloped in the heady fragrance of love and joy.

This is not a plant that we immediately think of as a medicine, but it has been used with great acclaim as an asthma remedy in the past, highly recommended by herbalists down through the ages as "it is fitting

84

that a conserve made of the flowers of it were kept in every gentlewoman's house as a cure for asthma." The flowers are rich in salicylic acid, which is what aspirin is made from, and they are also antispasmodic and expectorant, making sense as to why the herb had a reputation for headaches, croup and bronchitis and as a sovereign remedy for asthma. It is also applicable for headaches of a nervous kind. I have not used it for this purpose, but it seems that the flowers are antispasmodic to the voluntary as well as the involuntary muscles, as the herbalists of the 16th and 17th centuries suggested steeping the flowers in oil and leaving this to extract in the sun; it would then be used as a lovely massage oil "for those bodies… with cramps and convulsions."

Honeysuckle Cough Honey

Simply collect the flowers in the evening when they open and push them into a jar of runny honey until the jar is packed full. Strain this after four days and repeat three times. Take a teaspoon as required.

Recently Chinese scientists proved the powerful antiviral properties of the Japanese honeysuckle, *Lonicera japonica*. The papers lauded it as 'the new virological penicillin' and proclaimed that it may be effective against Ebola, and "this is where they should have been looking when researching anti-Ebola medicines."[20] Imagine if African farmers could grow and harvest the plants for the pharmaceutical companies to produce this new virological penicillin? So many problems could be solved, if it weren't for the inevitable industrial greed.

The Lime or Linden Tree (*Tilea cordata*)

In early July, the billowing linden trees pop into blossoms of little green pompoms. This is a rather subtle affair with the lime green flowers being of modest appearance, but their perfume is utterly sublime. To stand beneath one of these giants in the late afternoon sunshine is an awe-inspiring and almost narcotic experience. The warm air is delicately infused with an intoxicating perfume and the tree is alive with the drowsy humming of bees. Let go of your thoughts and allow your senses to open and become submerged in the trance-like fragrant hum. Your mind merges with the utter joy of the life force around you. Feel the magic of natural flow take over your body as you slowly work your way round the lowest branches, picking little flowers and filling your small basket with your harvest, listening to the drone of the bees, the rustle of the leaves, feeling the breeze on your face, filling your lungs with the perfumed air...

Now, look up and see the hundreds of thousands of flowers. This tree is like a cumulonimbus cloud of fragrant blossoms feeding the bees. People pray for abundance in life but look at the abundance of flowers on this single tree! One could not possibly pick them all. The flowers feed the bees, and they give us their honey in turn. We should align ourselves with Mother Nature and remember how to appreciate her gifts.

Linden blossoms are very relaxing. Popular in France as a tea (tilleul), they are taken to help promote sleep. The flowers are absolutely safe to give to restless children as an infusion with a little honey and equally effective for adults. They help to relieve high blood pressure by relaxing the mind and gently dilating the blood vessels. Lime flower baths were also once used for hysteria, for nervous vomiting or palpitations.

Relaxing Herbal Bath

We can make a beautifully fragrant and relaxing bath by collecting a double handful of linden blossoms, another of lemon balm (melissa) and another of lavender from the garden. Add all the herbs to a large teapot and cover with boiling water for about five minutes, then add them to the bath and relax.

Hedge Woundwort (*Stachys sylvatica*)

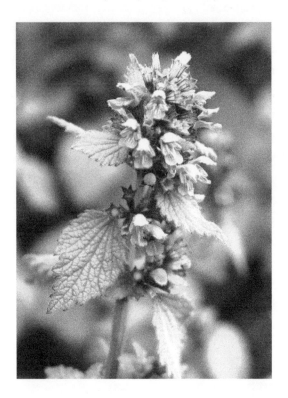

Hedge woundwort is a pretty but malodorous plant, identifiable in the hedges and fields at this time of year by its small sage-like purple flowers and unpleasant smell. As the name suggests, it has enjoyed an enduring reputation as a herb to heal wounds.

The 17th century herbalist John Gerard says of it, "The leaves hereof stamped with hog's grease and applied unto greene wounds in the manner of a pultesse, heale them in short time and in such absolute manner, that it is hard for any that have not had the experience thereof to beleeve."

There is an interesting story about this plant and John Gerard. In the 1600s when Gerard wrote his herbal, the physicians were very prone to bragging about their wonderful selves, and Gerard was no better. Even though he was not a doctor, he clearly still considered himself to be a fabulous healer. Whilst out walking one day, he came across a peasant who had cut himself deeply to the bone with a scythe. Gerard tells us, "I offered to heal him for charity's sake [that is, for free]." However, the peasant declined, walking off into the hedgerow to collect a bunch of woundwort; he must have pulverised this between two stones and applied it directly to the wound as a poultice, then carried on scything. Gerard was both deeply outraged that his charity had been refused and fascinated at the effectiveness of the plant, and he thereafter named the plant clown's woundwort. Presumably, 'clown' referred to the peasant. Culpeper, the 17th century apothecary was also a marvellous braggart and refused to acknowledge Gerard; he wrote that he "knows not why it is referred to as clown's woundwort", but admits that "it is inferior to none" in its ability to heal wounds.

This is not a herb which medical herbalists use today but it has a very long history, and even before Gerard it was known as All Heal. As the herb stops bleeding and promotes the healing of tissues so splendidly, it makes a safe and excellent first aid ointment.

Woundwort Honey

Cut the herb early in July and bruise it in a mortar and pestle, then push it into a wide neck glass jar that has been sterilised, preferably by heat in the oven. Gently warm raw honey in a bain marie and then pour it over the bruised herb. Poke the honey with a chopstick or something similar to release air bubbles and then close the lid.

Leave the jar on a sunny windowsill for two to four weeks and then strain the honey. You can use this herbal honey for slow-to-heal wounds such as varicose leg ulcers, abscesses or burns. It is best to apply the honey generously to a bandage and then to dress the wound.

Wild Lettuce (*Lactuca virosa*)

In these times of high-speed living, achieving a quiet mind is finding sanctuary in a world of chaos. But we over-think, and when it comes to bedtime our minds can have difficulty quietening down. For maintenance of health and a cheerful disposition, restful sleep is so important. Spending time in the hedgerows is a wonderful way to counter-balance the stressful pace of life, but few of us have the time to indulge in that pleasant pastime often enough to ensure a peaceful sleep every night. Nonetheless, the kindly hedgerows continue to help us by providing soporific wild lettuce.

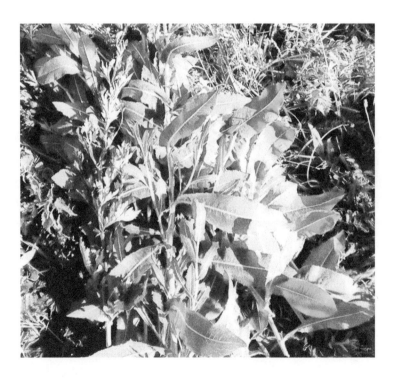

Lactuca comes from the Latin word for milk, 'lac'. If we snap the stem of wild lettuce we find a white milky sap oozes out which contains a substance called lactucarium, commonly known as lettuce opium. Herbalists use this herb as a gentle sedative and mild pain reliever. In large doses, it is said that the herb is slightly narcotic, promoting a feeling of euphoria, and there are records of this herb being used in the old witches' salves or flying ointments. In the medieval times of the witch burnings, one woman who believed she had flown through the air found herself in the courts charged with practising witchcraft. This would have been a terrifying ordeal because if she had been found guilty she would have been hanged or burned. She must have been fairly well off though because she had a clever lawyer who challenged the judge by enquiring whether there was a law against flying, and she luckily escaped with her neck intact.

The hippies of the 1960s also loved to promote this herb as a 'legal high'. I am amazed that they were so keen on it because it is also used to suppress sexual passion. For those who needed to distract themselves from such thoughts, instructions included washing oneself in cold lettuce tea and then wrapping the leftover spiky, cold and dripping leaves around one's genitals, which is probably enough to dampen anyone's ardour. This is not a herb that I would encourage the layperson to use, but as medical herbalists we use it in careful doses to encourage a peaceful sleep. It is especially helpful when pain is interrupting sleep or when one has a dry irritable coughs keeping them awake at night.

It is difficult to know how to put this but, in my opinion, the spirit of plants interacts with our minds. It has been well established by now that plants have memory and intelligence, so I don't believe that it is too unreasonable to consider that they may influence our thoughts, as I describe here…

One day, I decided to go hunting for wild lettuce and walked into the water meadows looking for it, but I could only see one or two plants. Because it is decent manners to thank the plant for its sacrifice and to leave much more than you take, I took very little of these few plants but thanked them gratefully. Quite soon, right in front of my eyes quite a few more wild lettuce plants appeared; I laughed and thanked them even more heartily, all the time telling them how wonderful they are. Then I noticed that the more I thanked the more plants I could see, until before my amazed eyes I had an entire meadow full of wild lettuce, where just a few minutes previously I could see only one or two.

It made me think of the effect of gratitude. As one thanks, one projects a loving vibration that is infallibly returned in greater abundance, so in being grateful we initiate a clear and definite cycle of positive energy in our lives that can have an immediate or delayed effect. I left the meadows that day with my basket overflowing with wild lettuce and my heart overflowing with wonder and gratitude for wild weeds.

Horsetail (*Equisetum arvense*)

Along with nettles, this plant is another plague of the gardener. If only the gardener understood that rather than tossing away handfuls of the weeds she could be drinking an infusion of both, then growing abundant hair and strong nails as well as toning her varicose veins. Indeed, both nettles and horsetail are rich in silica, which strengthens collagen, the matrix holding our tissues together.

Medical herbalists use this herb for all conditions related to weak collagen. The silica is water soluble and available to the body to use as a mineral. We use horsetail to strengthen breaking nails, weak veins such as varicose veins and piles, brittle hair and prolapses, and I would suggest that it may make an excellent anti-wrinkle herb too.

Women who struggle with mild urinary incontinence after childbirth may find they have more control over their bladder if they took horsetail. The herb can be used to help repair damaged tissue in the joints, and those with the wear-and-tear type of arthritis may find benefit. It can be used to improve recovery after surgery. In Scotland, horsetail was used to speed the healing of wounds by boiling the stems and leaves in water and then washing wounds in the infusion. Leg ulcers, which are slow to heal, can also be treated in the same way.

As herbalists, we may even use it in the cases of weak lungs, which have been damaged by chronic bronchitis. When a person coughs vigorously for a long period of time, the delicate lung tissue rips, in time progressing towards the severe damage of emphysema. *Equisetum* cannot repair the damage but it can strengthen the remaining lung tissue so that the damage is limited and the progress towards emphysema is delayed as long as possible. We might include herbs to thin the mucus in our prescription, such as *Plantago lanceolata*, and aid expectoration with *Inula helenium* to further help reduce the coughing.

Richard Mabey (Flora Britannica, Chatto & Windus 1996) relates how this plant has antifungal properties and that it is more successful for rose mildew than the proprietary fungicides. Try boiling the tops in water to make a strong infusion, then use the tail-like stems dipped into the cooled infusion to flick the liquid onto rose bushes, or strain it and use a normal spraying device.

One of its old names, scrubby-plant, tells us how traditionally the plant has been used as an abrasive agent for smoothing arrow heads, by housekeepers of old for scrubbing pots and pans and by watchmakers for shining brass and silver. If you drag the plant through your hands you will notice that it feels rough and tough enough, for example, to clean tarnished old candlesticks.

Vervain (*Verbena officinalis*)

Known as the Magician's Plant or the Wizard's Herb, this was one of the favourite herbs of the ancient Druids, although there does not seem to be clear evidence as to exactly why they revered it so much. Through the ages of history it has been known as a sacred herb; we see the ancient Druids use it in their lustral waters, thought to bring about purification, good luck and said to drive away all poisons. We must bear in mind that illness was perceived as 'flying venoms', then we see that vervain, by being said to drive away all poisons, was honoured with an implied title of panacea. The Romans used it as an alter plant where it was known as the Herba Sacra.

Others suggest that it opened 'the sight', the power of clairvoyant vision. We do know that it was one of the four sacred herbs of the Druids and that, when harvested, a libation of honey was offered to the plant. When I harvest my vervain, I leave a jar with remnants of honey and within two days the ants have cleaned it out. Perhaps the ants take the honey into the soil where the vervain roots can access the sugary solution. Even until recently, vervain seems to have retained its magical associations; only a few decades ago it was commonly hung around the neck on a white ribbon or within a black silk bag to promote general health for the wearer. Modern Druids use it as a herb to open us to the flow of the Awen (divine inspiration).

Therapeutically, vervain focuses its actions on the liver and the nervous system — as does betony, but there is a subtle difference. Betony is more protective whilst vervain is more opening.

When vervain is taken, one feels a sense of peacefulness and slight euphoria. This gently opens the mind up to the flow of Awen, the magical flow of inspiration. The Awen flows through all of life and opening oneself up to the Awen allows us to feel joy and express our creativity in our own unique ways, our gifts to the universe. For instance, for me it can occur when working with herbs or when in the wilderness. For others it may be through music or creating something, which in the mere doing opens the flow of universal peace, love and joy. This sense of flow happens when we stop thinking and just allow our natural inspiration and creativity to download.

We all can tap into Awen because it is available to everyone, but sometimes we are too preoccupied or over-analysing with the left brain. Vervain slows us down to a more natural rhythm so that we can engage with the Awen. When we restore the balance between the analytical left brain and the creative right brain, we connect with the person we really are; and the conditions for which vervain is so famously helpful such as depression, melancholy and hysteria, can fade away. As a medical herbalist, I use vervain to calm the over-wrought mind and to bring comfort and peace to a person. We say that vervain is as comforting as a mother's hug.

The bitter principals of the herb stimulate the liver to flush bile, helping to relieve liver congestion; hence its fame as a herb for jaundice. Verbena is also weakly oestrogenic, helping to promote milk flow in the new mother, possibly by also relaxing her. Later on in years, when she struggles with the menopause, it will also calm her and support her declining oestrogen levels.

The ancients were very specific about how herbs were to be collected, the time of harvest, by whom they should be harvested and how that person must approach the herb. Sometimes the herb may only be collected when the person was wearing white and walking unshod following a lustral bath. Frequently the instruction was that the plant may not be collected with the use of iron. Other instructions might include only plucking with the left hand or not looking over the shoulder as the herb is being harvested. In the case of vervain, it was to be collected at the dark of the moon, when Sirius was rising. The plant was cut with a sickle using the right hand. The left hand raised the herb to the skies and then a libation of honey was poured in gratitude over the earth. By comparison, this makes the mechanical harvesting of herbal medicines seem so brutal and sacrilegious.

Figwort (*Scrophularia nodosa*)

This is a hedgerow plant that seems to have become largely forgotten and even herbalists do not use it very often. As its name implies, scrophularia has been primarily employed in the past to treat scrofula, aka the King's Evil. This is a dreadful disease caused by the tuberculosis bacterium, resulting in massively enlarged glands in the neck and other parts which burst and exude pus, terribly deforming of the face and neck. It was believed that the king had the power to cure the disease simply by his touch – not a job that a king would look forward to, I should think.

This plant of ditches and bogs seems in the past to have had an affinity for the neck and throat, where amongst its many names are throatwort; the Romans called it cervicaria, after the cervical vertebrae in the neck. If you look at the roots of figwort, you will observe that they are nodular, suggesting, according to The Doctrine of Signatures, that the plant's gifts are in the clearing of glandular infections and strengthening weak veins such as varicose veins or piles, which were known as figs, hence the name.

As a modern medical herbalist, I use this plant when treating glandular fever, persistent tonsillitis or breast lumps, swelling of the testicles or chronic viral infections where the glands surrounding the neck are painfully enlarged. We also commonly use the plant with burdock and other cleansing herbs to clear skin conditions such as eczema, abscesses, pussy ulcers or psoriasis.

Evening Primrose (*Oenothera biennis*)

It first occurred to me that this plant can and should be used to balance female hormones as a herb, rather than as the encapsulated oil, when a young woman from Poland started talking to me about how they use it in Eastern Europe. The eastern Europeans are much more in touch with their hedgerow herbs than we are in the western parts. She told me that they simply eat the seeds, which makes complete sense because the seeds produce the famous evening primrose oil.

Evening primrose is a plant of the moon. Her petals open between 6 and 7 p.m., hence the name, and once opened the flower looks like a full moon, emitting a delicate fragrance. The petals themselves actually shine at night, again bringing to mind the gentle luminosity of the moon. The moon being a feminine planet suggests to us that we should tune our attention towards the possibilities of women's healing. It is indeed well known that evening primrose oil is used successfully to ease pre-menstrual tension, breast pain and menopausal symptoms. The omega-rich oils soften dry skin and condition brittle hair and nails. It is less well known that the American Cherokee drink a tea from the root to help lose weight.

Pliny, among others, refers to this plant as 'a happiness-maker'. It is interesting to note that the seeds are rich in tryptophan, which converts to serotonin, our 'happy hormone'. If you would like to try using the seeds yourself, you will need to harvest them in the autumn, dry them in an airing cupboard and grind them over porridge or into a smoothie. Omega oils turn rancid very quickly once exposed to the air, so I recommend grinding and using them immediately. A pepper grinder would be the perfect instrument.

The oils from evening primrose can be used to help prevent blood clotting, to protect arteries from hardening, as an anti-inflammatory agent for conditions such as arthritis and for dry itchy skin conditions such as eczema and psoriasis. In these cases, the oil capsules are probably more effective.

Before EPO became famous, the whole plant was used primarily to soothe the stomach by acting as a relaxing antispasmodic. The Doctrine of Signatures sees the round yellow flower as the yellow solar plexus chakra. It is particularly indicated for those who have eaten badly for years so that their gastric mucosa has become inflamed with accumulated toxins. Evening primrose herb will help to reduce the inflammation whilst gently and slowly clearing the congested liver. Traditionally the leaves and roots were also used for spasmodic conditions such as asthma and whooping cough.

The relaxing effect of the plant is particularly appropriate for those people who are suffering from adrenal burnout, where the body and mind are exhausted but the nervous system is highly agitated. These people are frequently both depressed and anxious, but they cannot get off the hamster wheel and have lost the ability to relax and open up to the joy of life. Their mental and emotional being feels tight, brittle and malfunctioning, and so soon enough the body breaks down. The herb allows the person to relax, then revitalises and rebalances the mind, body and spirit.

The evening primrose plant seems to be another one of the many hated weeds, but this is something I find difficult to understand as it is such a beautiful plant and, to my mind, equally as charming as hollyhocks. However, if you do have too many in your garden, be aware that the root was a popular vegetable in the 18th century. The roots, which look like small parsnips, can easily be pulled up. Rather than wasting them, try them as a new vegetable.

Corn Poppies (*Papaver rhoeas*)

With the increase in organic farming, corn poppies have begun to steal back into the fields; what a relief it is to see their brilliant red petals splashed against the wheat fields, breaking the monotony and running wildness into the regimented rows.

Poppies take us back to the Great War, reminding us of delicate lives now blown away. The flowers suggest life and love is as fragile and beautiful as a poppy petal. Before the war they grew with the wheat and during the war they became the symbol of lives cut too short and so precious. So we look at each spindly stem and paper-fine petals with a mixture of sadness at their brief flowering and yet, for this, we treasure each blossom all the more, as we should with all the loves in our lives, for life is fragile and our loved ones are to be treasured.

As always, nature is compassionate. If the poppy is associated with pain, it is also the reliever of pain. The corn poppy is much milder in its medical action than the opium poppy, but it still has a long history giving relief from pain and insomnia. The petals, turned into a syrup, may be taken for pain relief of any kind, to give peaceful sleep or to sooth a hacking cough, and in the past it was particularly used for the sharp pain of pleurisy.

The women who worked the fields knew that steeping a few petals in warmed milk would ensure that their babies slept through the night. A common country remedy was to crush and cook a few fresh seed heads in pigs' grease as a pain relieving unguent. Poppies were always to be found in cottage gardens because mothers knew that they could bring pain relief to their entire family just by decocting a few poppy heads in the kitchen.

For some reason that I cannot understand, people always seem to have feared plants and wilderness. When I trawl through old herbals, I see so many superstitions related to plants and flowers, including fears and horrors... 'If you touch a poppy and the petals fall off, then you are more likely to be struck by lightning.' 'If they were gathered and placed near the ear, then you will suffer a violent attack of earache.' 'If placed near the eyes then they will cause blindness or produce warts.' There have been long lists of the likely dangers of handling poppies. I have always loved poppies and have never been struck by lightning or suffered violent earache, I can still see just fine and I don't have warts.

It may be possible that mugwort and poppies were used in the ancient sleep temples such as the ruin found in Lydney Park, Gloucestershire. The temple is dedicated to Nodens, the Celtic god of dreaming (hence the Land of Nod), of healing, the sea, war, dogs and hunting. The vague information that we have about these sleep temples is that they were always associated with mineral springs, had a large bath house attached and small cells where the seeker spent the night. Beneath the temples were large pits filled with snakes, fed by means of a chute.

It seems that the pilgrim arrived at the temple seeking guidance from the deities in the form of a dream. The first therapeutic step may have involved offering a sacrifice to Nodens or another god or goddess, followed by a purification bath. The purifying lustral bath was a deep, warm mineral water bath in which specific herbs have been steeped. After this, there may also have been chanting and fasting to promote an altered state of consciousness. Murals show images of poppy seed heads, and it is likely that the sick person was given a draft of poppies and possibly mugwort, before being taken to their warm sleeping chamber, where specially trained healing priests watched over them. Upon awakening, the priest – more of an ancient psychoanalyst than a herbalist – was available to help the pilgrim interpret their dreams, thus to obtain a diagnosis or prognosis. The belief would have been that the dreams were messages from the gods and they would be received with reverence and interpreted with great respect.

But what of the snakes in the pit below the temple? As they slithered over each other, they would have created a humming noise, which may have generated a specific healing vibration to instigate lucid dreaming; or perhaps the snakes symbolised renewal as they shed their skins and appeared rejuvenated.

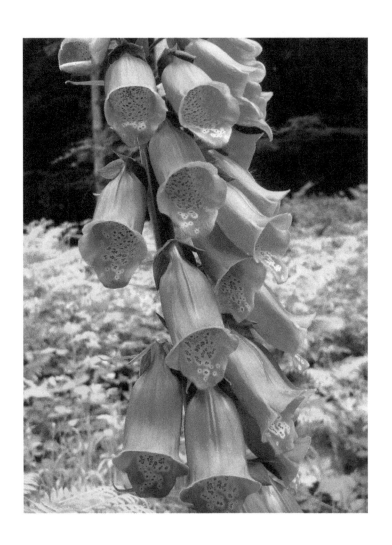

August

Lughnasadh and the first harvest. The sun has ripened the crops, and the Sun God has transferred his strength to the seeds. The god of the harvest, popularly known as John Barleycorn, is cut down or sacrificed to the land, to provide abundant food for the people.

In very ancient times, the king was literally sacrificed and his blood was sprinkled on the land to ensure fertility. Later that ritual gave way to the making of corn dollies and bread to celebrate the bounty of the land and to give thanks to the Sun God for giving his strength. This is the time of abundance.

Burdock (*Arctium lappa*)

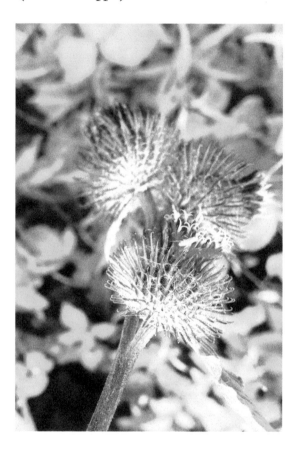

Big voluptuous burdock, the most handsome plant in the hedge-row. Stroke his leaves and it feels like you are stroking the ears of a green elephant. The burrs that knot into any nearby dog's fur seem to have provided humans with plenty of entertainment over the centu-ries. There is an old Cornish story that the piskies (Cornish faeries) amused themselves at night by riding colts furiously around the fields and tangling their manes with burrs.

Children used to play a game where burrs were thrown onto the backs of their friends. If the burrs stuck they had an admirer but if the burrs soon fell off then the affection would be short-lived. Perhaps the person who invented Velcro had played this game as a child and was inspired by the seeds, which hook so successfully onto clothing that in the past burdock was also called beggars' buttons.

In Lothian, Scotland, there is the annual tradition of the Burryman, a local chap dressed in overalls completely covered in burrs and flowers. He walks through the town receiving gifts and greetings from the locals and in turn bringing good fortune. Some suggest that he embodies the Green Man, whilst others suggest the burrs hook and take away all evil influences, thus cleansing the town of bad luck.

Interestingly, herbalists are very fond of using this herb as a deep tissue-cleansing herb. Many diseases are caused by toxic accumulations or are the result of obstruction to the natural elimination system. Burdock is our go-to plant, digging out the toxins and then eliminating them via the liver and bowels.

Detoxifying the body effectively and safely needs to be done slowly. When the body ingests a toxin, it packs the poison away safely in the fat cells until it can be eliminated. If we continue to eat junk food, breathe in polluted air, drink oestrogenated water and so on, our bodies have a hard time cleaning up; so the toxins accumulate in the cells. But releasing them too quickly can cause a toxic overload in the blood and too much for the liver and kidneys to deal with. Thus it is important to support the liver and kidneys first, so that they are in a good position to separate the toxins from the blood and eliminate them via the stools or urine.

Herbs such as dandelion root and milk thistle help the liver, whereas dandelion leaf, cleavers and pellitory-of-the-wall support the kidneys. Then it is important to encourage the blood to flush the tissues, so one would include yarrow and horseradish. Only then can we use our detox herbs such as nettles, ground elder and burdock to dig the toxins out of the cells and release them into the blood stream, to be delivered to the liver and kidneys for elimination.

Burdock root also has a mild laxative and diuretic effect, in this way encouraging the elimination of the toxins from the liver and kidneys; isn't nature absolutely wonderful? The plant pulls the toxins from deep in the cells and then stimulates its release from the two major organs of elimination. There is no drug invented that could hope to achieve so much. Traditionally in Europe, we use only the root, which is the detoxifying part of the plant. But the leaf is a natural antibiotic and the seeds are rich in nourishing oils, so in our apothecaries we use the seeds, leaf and root in our tincture, making it very appropriate for eczema, acne and psoriasis.

Burdock provides some culinary surprises. The young stalks can be eaten as a vegetable, similar to asparagus. To do this, peel the stalk leaving only the soft core. Boil or steam this until soft and serve it with melted butter or hollandaise sauce, or try the stems battered and fried like tempura and served with sweet chilli or soy sauce. The root is eaten as a vegetable called gobo in Japan.

Japanese Gobo

To make this dish, we need to dig the root in autumn, peel it and cut it into thin matchsticks. Marinate them for two hours in soy sauce, then just cover them with water in a pan and simmer until the water has completely evaporated and the soy sauce has concentrated into the root, being careful not to allow it to burn. Serve with a drizzle of sesame oil and a sprinkling of sesame seeds.

Yarrow (*Achillea millefolium*)

Yarrow is not so much a plant of the hedgerow but more a herb of the sort of rough meadows where horses graze contentedly in a sea of buttercups, red clover and yarrow. We are told that the god

Achilles used it to staunch the bleeding wounds of his soldiers, so it was known in ancient times as herba militaris, the herb of soldiers. The species name of this plant means 'thousand leaf', referring to the greatly divided leaf resembling a feather. Yet again, our Doctrine of Signatures indicates to us how the plant is used medically. When we observe the feathery leaf and note its tiny segments, this clearly suggests the fine capillaries of our peripheral circulatory system upon which this plant acts.

Herbalists believe that plants have an innate intelligence and their actions are amphoteric: in other words, they do what is needed in the body. If we read the texts concerning yarrow, we learn that it both stops bleeding and promotes bleeding, which could lead to some confusion! Leave it to the yarrow to decide what is required. Plants have been working on human bodies for hundreds of thousands of years and they know just what to do.

One of its old names is nosebleed, and here we see the contradictory nature of the herb. It is suggested that if you have a nosebleed, you should roll it into a ball and stuff it up your nose to stop the bleed: but also, if you have a headache, then roll it up your nose and it will cause profuse bleeding which will decongest the head... I presume that the last recipe came from the days when bloodletting was fashionable. We tend to use the herb now to support poor circulation to the peripheries in cases such as Raynaud's Disease and varicose ulcers. We also find it very helpful for women who have poor pelvic circulation, which results in a stagnant blood flow and painful periods with blood clots. Yarrow gently improves the uterine blood circulation and eases the passing of menstrual blood.

Yarrow is also very helpful for relieving high blood pressure. We live in such hectic times, with many people racing about achieving everything they can. Their poor nervous systems are like tightly coiled springs, as are the muscles of their blood vessels. Combining yarrow with linden blossom or vervain helps the person to relax, allowing the tiny muscles surrounding the blood vessels to relax; the blood vessels dilate so that the pressure in the circulatory system normalises to a healthier level.

Yarrow has famously been used as a diaphoretic too, in the times when people did not have aspirin to reduce a high temperature. Diaphoretics promote perspiration, which cools the body. A well-known herbal remedy for a high temperature is to make an infusion of yarrow, elderflowers and peppermint. The yarrow and elderflowers dilate the capillaries, promoting perspiration and cooling the fever. Yarrow is appropriate for any condition where the circulation is inadequate due to tightness of the capillaries. If poor circulation is caused by a weak heart then hawthorn needs to be considered, but there is no reason why yarrow would not be useful too depending on the situation.

Herbs have such a strong association with spells, and the most prolific spells must be those of young ladies trying to divine their future husbands. Yarrow is incorporated into many love spells, which include picking yarrow off a young man's grave at midnight, tying the sprig to the thigh and then getting into bed backwards whilst saying goodnight to the yarrow and entreating it to reveal the name of one's true love. I read a story of an old lady who knew someone who had performed this spell, and she related in an awed voice that he had come to her in the night (presumably in a dream) and revealed his name. In due course, she married two men by that same name! So it must have worked.

A lazier option involves tickling the inside of the nose with yarrow whilst chanting, "Yarroway, yarroway, bear a white blow; if my love loves me, my nose will bleed now." Carrying yarrow in the wedding bouquet was considered a guarantee of seven years of married bliss, but after this, I suppose, a renewal spell had to be concocted.

Betony (*Stachys betonica*)

"Sell your coat and buy betony" is an old Italian proverb. Such was the value of this plant that for centuries it was considered a panacea for most illnesses. It was grown in all the physic gardens of the apothecaries and monasteries, with some plants continuing to flourish on the sites despite the institutions having falling into ruin long ago. Our herbs really do give many clues to the past. As a wild plant, it is found amongst the grasses and mints of riverbanks and along the shady edges of meadows. It acts as a refrigerant herb, cooling an overheated head, the central nervous system and the liver. Betony has a particular affinity for afflictions of the head and is an effective herb for headaches, bad dreams, dizziness, vertigo, anxiety, hysteria and neuralgia.

The old books say that it should be gathered on a Thursday in the month of August, without the use of iron. Not using iron is quite a common instruction for the gathering of herbs. Those who are in touch with the spirits of the plants tell us that the elementals abhor iron. Why? Maybe the troubles of the world began with the Iron Age. Man seems to have lived in relative peace and balance with the Earth until iron started carving up the land for crops, mining for more iron and chopping down forest to melt it into arrowheads and swords. Iron is harsh against soft materials like wood and soil, providing the means for the Earth's resources to be over harvested and fought over. Alas, we always want more.

This herb was a favourite of those ale-drinking Saxons who would chew a leaf of betony before a drunken party to prevent a hangover – there's a good tip! Being a bitter herb, betony stimulates the liver to flush bile into the colon and out via the bowels. In this way it helps the organ to cope with an overload of alcohol. On the other hand, some herbals say that eating the leaf is quite intoxicating, so perhaps they were just pre-empting the party? One way or another, betony has been favoured as a cure for hangovers for hundreds of years.

An interesting quality of betony, which I still use today, is that it was believed to keep away evil spirits, and was said to "shield people against visions and dreams... driving away devils and despair." Vapour baths of the herb were prescribed for "those that be ferfull", and I have found it helpful for those who feel vulnerable, under psychic attack or waking with night terrors, or even feel they want protection from 'energy vampires' or those with unwholesome energies. Whether you chose to believe in this or not, betony and St John's wort have, for a very long time, been regarded as herbs of protection against negative energies; I have certainly found them to be very consoling for those who do feel vulnerable to such influences.

The old manuscripts relate over forty-seven uses of the plant and conclude that there are even more besides. Modern herbalists tend mostly to use betony for conditions of the liver, nervous system and the head as explained above. Older herbalists highly recommended this plant for tuberculosis, jaundice, palsy, convulsions, acne, cancerous sores, gravel, cough, gout, dropsy, bites of serpents and mad dogs, and as a herbal tobacco. This is only my personal opinion, but I think that we, modern herbalists, have quite a feeble knowledge of plant medicine when compared to the herbalists of the olden days...

The physician to the Roman Emperor Augustus, addressed the plant thus: "Betony, you who were discovered first by Aesculapius or by Chiron the centaur, hear my prayer. I implore you, herb of strength, by Him who ordered your creation and ordered that you should be useful for a multitude of remedies, kindly help in making these seven and forty remedies."

Hemp Agrimony (*Eupatorium cannabinum*)

This is a common hedgerow plant, entirely ignored by medical herbalists today, and I must urge you not to use this plant internally; I have never used it, nor can I account for its safe use. It contains certain alkaloids that may damage the liver if taken on a regular basis or in large doses. Despite its potentially liver damaging alkaloids, hemp agrimony has a long reputation as a treatment for congested livers or jaundice. Still, we have to be careful, so consider this for information only. Bear in mind that most people who used herbs for medicine were sensible, employing small doses, and thus were able to enjoy the benefits of the plant. Anything, when prescribed in massive quantities, is potentially poisonous.

The leaves contain constituents that act on the kidneys as a diuretic, and in doing so the plant helps to alleviate excess fluids in the body; indeed, the herb was used in times gone by for swollen feet and as a blood cleanser. The leaves, when boiled to a paste, are said to cure swollen testicles and I would think that this would be helpful for all swollen glands, including mastitis.

Like its better known sister plant *Eupatorium perfoliatum*, which we do use frequently during the winter, this herb has been recorded as very helpful for the fevers of influenza or severe colds where there the persons feels hot and cold, sweating and chilled. Both plants are used for congested lungs and coughs. *Eupatorium perfoliatum* is used for those `flu symptoms where one aches to the bones, shivering with fevers and chills, and where a person has difficulty breathing. Looking at the past reputation of hemp agrimony, it appears to have very similar properties.

The leaves of *Eupatorium cannabinum* are rich in volatile oils and polysaccharides which have immune stimulating actions, and so we can understand why this herb gives quick relief for feverish influenza and possibly may play a role in future cancer treatments. Indeed, a study in 2014 found it to have the ability to kill colon cancer cells, meriting its further investigation as a chemotherapeutic agent[21].

Culpeper tells us, "I hold it inferior to but few herbs..." He states that it helps with cachexia, a wasting of the body or evil disposition of the body, which may or may not relate to cancer. He also notes that it breaks up infected abscesses, clears jaundice, relieves an enlarged spleen, and breaks fevers. Here we see the association with glandular and infectious conditions.

Red Clover (*Trifolium pratense*)

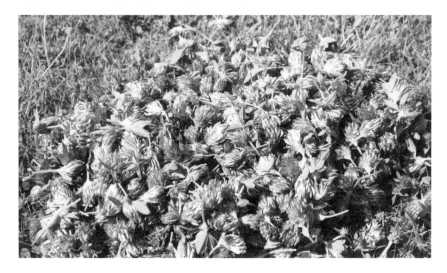

Red clover is another 'weed' ruthlessly pulled out by gardeners without realising the value that it holds for us. In the past, red clover had a strong reputation as a cure for skin cancer, when it was boiled down into a dark mass and the poultice applied over the affected area. It was also used, as we still do today, for the treatment of eczema and psoriasis. Usually, we prescribe it as an infusion or as part of a tincture formula for its blood-cleansing properties, but the plant also contains allantoin, which promotes the healing and growth of healthy skin tissue.

We accumulate toxins from a poor diet, by living in cities, drinking too much alcohol or coffee and so on. In order to stay healthy and vibrant, our wise body knows that it needs to eliminate the toxins; but if the liver is sluggish due to a fatty diet or too much alcohol consumption, or the bowels are constipated, or the kidneys are burdened under a heavy protein diet, they struggle to get rid of the accumulated toxins through these routes. The toxins are then delivered to the next organ of elimination, which is the skin, and this is when we see breakouts of eczema, boils or psoriasis. It is just the body trying to get rid of an excessive toxic burden. However, the above skin disorders can also be symptoms of a person under too much stress.

As herbalists, our job is to use herbs to assist the body in its natural function by opening up the pathways of elimination, through supporting the liver, the kidneys and the circulation and also by cleansing the cells themselves with, in this case, red clover. It would not be wise only to use a blood-cleanser without making sure that the major organs of elimination are working well. If the toxins that have been stored in the cells are released into the bloodstream, and the liver or kidneys are under-functioning, they cannot perform their job adequately so consequently there is a flare-up of the skin condition. This is not uncommon and, when it happens, we have to stop the blood-cleanser and go back to the liver and kidney support until they are ready to remove the toxins safely.

Red clover is a bronchial antispasmodic herb with expectorant qualities, and can be supportive in the treatment of bronchitis and whooping cough. Combining it with marshmallow leaves or root and liquorice as a herbal tea would soothe the rough, barking cough.

Today it is better known as a phyto-oestrogenic herb and is used as a natural substitute for HRT by women with menopausal symptoms. The whole herb is rich in isoflavones, which are the phyto- (plant) oestrogens. Phyto-oestrogens are weakly oestrogenic and there is much controversy over whether they may be used by those who have had oestrogen-driven cancers. Trawling through several research papers, the results seem to suggest that red clover is actually protective against oestrogen-driven cancers. The weak phyto-oestrogens dock into the oestrogen receptor sites of the body and occupy these sites, blocking the more aggressive cancer-stimulating oestrogens from acting.

In the days when folk believed so strongly in elves and faeries that they looked with incredulity at anyone who denied their existence, the four-leaf clover was considered lucky because it had the virtue of being able to dissolve faery spells. On the other hand, four grains of wheat wrapped inside a cloverleaf enabled the wearer to see elves and goblins. I am unsure why they would want to see the elves and goblins, for these beings were greatly feared.

Brambles (*Rubus fructicosus*)

A forgotten name for the long, thorny canes of brambles is 'lawyers' because of the difficulty one has of extricating oneself from their grasp! Nonetheless, despite thorny scratches, one of the great joys of the late English summer is spending a warm Sunday afternoon meandering along the hedgerows collecting blackberries. This annual ritual represents one of the last vestiges of foraging for food in Britain. What a treat it is to come home with a hoard of berries and turn them into a blackberry crumble to be savoured after dinner with double cream or, sinfully, for breakfast the next day.

Bruce, the fat-bottomed chocolate labrador who often accompanies my hedgerow forays, loves to munch the berries that I toss him, topping up his anti-oxidants. It is the dark colouring of the fruit that provides rather amazing health benefits. Natural chemicals called anthrocyanins and ellagic acid are highly anti-oxidant, anti-inflammatory and have anti-tumour effects. Clinical trials repeatedly have shown that these constituents in blackberries inhibit the growth and spread of cancer cells.

The anthrocyanins found in these common and humble fruits are also helpful in conditions such as diabetes, where the high blood sugars damage the capillary walls in the retina of the eye, leading to blindness. Anthrocyanins strengthen blood vessel walls, protecting the capillaries from damage, and they are particularly helpful in conditions such as diabetic retinopathy, piles, varicose veins, or simply where the blood vessel walls have become weak and the person bruises easily.

The berries are packed with vitamin C. A lovely way of naturally boosting your immune system through the winter is to collect the berries, rinse them and, once dried, pop them straight into the freezer. Every morning, you can blend a handful of frozen blackberries and a teaspoon of elderberries with rice milk and a banana into a delicious health-promoting purple smoothie. Another option is to dry them in a cool oven then grind them into a powder, which can be added to a smoothie or sprinkled over porridge.

The leaves are rich in astringent tannins. Astringency contracts and dries tissues, and this action is valuable in inflammatory conditions where the tissues become boggy and engorged with fluids. Astringency also disables bacteria by 'cold-cooking' the bacterial proteins, making this plant ideal as a gargle for inflamed sore throats or bleeding gums and as a tea to relieve diarrhoea and inflamed intestines.

Another old name for blackberries is 'hind berry' because at certain times of year the female deer will eat the plant. I noticed in my old herb garden that once a year the deer leapt the surrounding fence and severely pruned my roses... Women have known for generations that drinking raspberry leaf tea encourages stronger and more effective labour contractions. Roses, raspberries and blackberries all belong to the rosacea family of plants, so I suspect that the hinds must have been using the blackberry or rose leaves for similar purposes.

The blackberry bush demonstrates, once again, Mother Nature's abundant generosity. Notice the enormous quantities of fruit produced: there is more than enough for everyone to enjoy their crumbles, tarts, jams and jellies with still plenty left over to fatten the birds and mice for the coming winter.

Sweet and Savoury Blackberry Crumble

Combine equal quantities of blackberries and peeled, chopped apples. Place them in a buttered ovenproof dish and sprinkle with cinnamon and demerara sugar. Add the odd clove or two, or even a sprig of rosemary if you wish.

In a separate bowl, mix equal portions of rolled oats and ground almonds, enough to cover the fruit. Then add some demerara sugar to taste but not too much. Now, to the oats and almonds add a handful of grated vintage cheddar cheese and then rub in sufficient fresh butter to form the crumbles. Sprinkle the crumble on top of the fruit so that the fruit is covered by nearly an inch of crumble.

Pop it in the oven and bake until the crumble has turned nicely brown and crunchy. The fruit will have cooked and gently caramelised at the edges. Serve warm with ice cream or double cream – and keep a little for breakfast!

White Deadnettle (*Lamium album*)

Deadnettle is a common plant found in cool areas and is an excellent example of the slyness of plants. Being soft and juicy, and having a low growth habit, it has no means of protecting itself against grazing animals save by pretending to be what it is not. By disguising itself as a stinging nettle, and then tucking itself in amongst the nettles, it hopes to be passed unnoticed!

There is an enchanting story about deadnettles, which tells us about the faeries that did not like getting their shoes wet as they danced in dewy meadows under the moonlight. Before dancing, they would put their shoes to one side, but the centipedes kept stealing them. So the faeries decided to hide their shoes in the nettle flowers, though first they had to cast a spell over the nettles to avoid being stung. Notice that if you pick a sprig of white deadnettle and turn it upside down, you will find a tiny pair of black shoes hidden neatly within each white flower...

Lamium is traditionally used by herbalists as 'a women's herb', mainly used to reduce heavy menstrual flow. Although deadnettle are not botanically related to stinging nettles, it is interesting that stinging nettles are also used to check the flow of excessive bleeding. If a woman does not have large fibroids or any other cause of excessive blood flow, then these two herbs can be combined very successfully to check the flow of heavy menstrual bleeding and rebuild the blood afterwards.

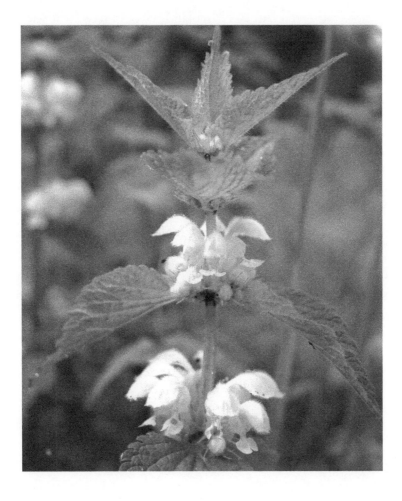

Heather (*Calluna vulgaris*)

Who hasn't bought a sprig of lucky heather from a London gypsy? Lucky heather seems to be a Highland belief and white heather is considered the luckiest, maybe because it is rare or maybe because a Scottish tradition tells us that it grows where the faeries have rested. According to Scottish tradition, white heather almost always features in bridal bouquets, presumably to bring luck to the couple.

Queen Victoria recorded on the 9th of September, 1872, while out for a drive with Brown, that he "espied a piece of white heather, and jumped off to pick it. No Highlander would pass by it without picking it, for it was considered to bring good luck."

The old Celts associated heather with the honeybee. The bees, by aligning themselves to the sun, travelled to the heather from the hive and were seen as messengers from the spirit world. In the Druid tradition, the bees are the creatures that bring heather nectar back to their hive through working as a community. The nectar is turned into honey, which is shared by all. Heather, by association, thus represents sweetness, celebration, sharing and community. Possibly this is why heather is considered lucky, for how much luckier can we be than when we share love and the sweetness in life, like the hives overflowing with heather honey?

For at least 4,000 years the resourceful Scots have materialised this sweetness by brewing heather ale. Excavations of a Neolithic settlement found evidence of an ale made from oats, barley, heather and meadowsweet, which sounds rather delicious. Robert Louis Stevenson celebrates its joys in his poem titled Heather Ale, which would cheer up any crisp and snowy Highland night:

"From the bonny bells of heather, they brewed a drink long syne,
was sweeter far than honey, was stronger far than wine."

The Picts were also known to make a sublime wine from heather flowers, which contained enough nectar to account for its sweetness. In the fourth century, Viking raiders massacred all people of a Shetland isle except for a father and son, who were spared only so that they could give those Norsemen their secret recipe. In the agonies of torture, the father agreed to tell them but only if they would first kill his son. Once the boy had died, the father triumphantly told the conquerors that he hadn't been convinced that his son could hold out, but he himself would never tell – and so his recipe went with him to his grave.

Until fairly recently, the Scottish people used to make mattresses and pillows from heather or, more simply, a sprig was placed under the pillow. I myself can attest that I have never slept so well as the night I slept out on the Highlands with springy heather as my mattress.

Heather has been used as a tea both to bring a restful sleep, for frayed nerves, and as a tonic to revive jaded spirits. I can find no good reason for not bringing back heather as an antidepressant medicine for nervous exhaustion in these times of extreme stress and anxiety. Today, modern herbalists rarely use heather as a medicine, but it is recorded in our formularies as useful for urinary tract infections, kidney stones and rheumatism, and was used as such by Brother Aloysius in 1901.

I remember once, riding horses across the Black Mountains in Wales with a friend of mine, and gazing at the glory of the lonely mountainsides absolutely covered in a cloak of magenta. On that windswept and desolate mountain with black storm clouds charging overhead, a ray of sunshine pierced through the darkness onto the heather and the colour was of an otherworldly beauty. The thick toffee-like heather honey always makes me smile when I remember the beauty of heather on those mountainsides and industrious bees who create the first sweetness humankind ever tasted.

September

At the autumn equinox we have the final harvest of the year. The last warmth of summer is gentle and nostalgic. The days are of equal length as the nights. This is a time when berries have ripened and the last of the herbs have been gathered. The work of the year is over, goals have been achieved, the harvest is in and we prepare for the colder days around the fire, eating the fat of the land, which we have worked hard to harvest. But even if we don't physically harvest any longer, we can still look at the hedgerow, noticing the abundance of fruits and nuts, and take some time to give thanks for our own harvest of the year.

This is a time of gratitude, when we can reflect on our blessings of the year: the money in the bank, our lovely home and the satisfaction we derive from our work and pleasures. A nice way to celebrate the harvest time is to make jam from hedgerow berries: we should remember to stir into the pot our gratitude to the land and the love we hold for those who will enjoy this jam. We could also make bird cakes for those little creatures that have to spend the winter out in the cold.

The Rowan Tree (*Sorbus aucuparia*)

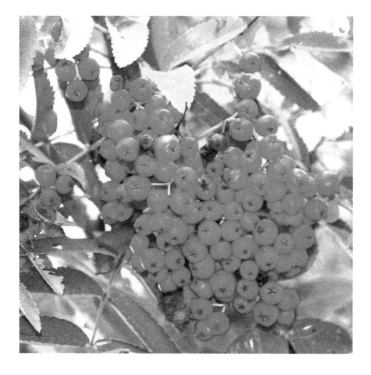

At this time of year, the rowan displays clusters of vibrant orange-red berries. This tree has a strong folk association with protection, particularly against witches and all evil things. In the past, it was common to find rowan trees, also known as mountain ash, planted outside a front door, or even to find rowan twigs formed into crosses and tied with sheep's wool or red thread. These talismans were hung over the doorways of houses, in barns, on horse's headbands and even tied to the tails of cows. An old saying tells us, "Rowan wood and red thread, makes the witches tremble in dread." Even today, some keep a rowan twig about their person for protection against negative influences or to shield against psychic or harmful energies.

In Scotland it was said that faeries live in the rowan tree and that these trees often protect the stone circles where faeries love to dance. Rowan berries are still used for protection, but latterly more against sore throats than witches! The berry, rich in vitamin C, is traditionally used to treat scurvy and, in modern times, to ease sore throats, tonsillitis and particularly for soothing hoarseness. Rowan berry syrup is highly valued by singers.

Caution: Rowan berry jelly is excellent to eat with fatty meat such as roast pork or sausages, but if you make your own please be aware that the seeds are poisonous, so make sure that they are strained from the warm jelly before bottling. The fruit itself is safe to eat and has a lovely wild flavour with a sharp tartness.

Rowan Berry Throat Syrup

Collect a large jam jar of the ripe berries and make a note of the berries' weight, then wash them well and just cover with boiling water. Add a stick of cinnamon and simmer for five minutes, then add one tablespoon of apple cider vinegar before straining, keeping the liquid.

Now to work out how much sugar to add: measure the quantity of liquid, then on a calculator divide the millilitres of liquid by 10 and then multiply that figure by 7. This is the quantity of sugar in grams to be dissolved into the warm rowan liquid. Store it in a sterilised glass bottle and, whenever you feel your throat is sore or scratchy, take a teaspoon four times a day for a maximum of three days.

Hedgerow Jelly

One of my personal favourite cold and 'flu protection methods is to use hedgerow jelly. This is my own rather unprofessional recipe, but it has a beautiful taste and is packed with antiviral and immune-enhancing plants. Included in this recipe are the antiviral elderberries and blackberries, mentioned in June and August respectively.

Near my home is an ancient wood in which grows a crab apple tree. I collect a few crab apples, some blackberries, elderberries, rowan berries and a few bay leaves. I drop the whole lot into a pot with a small amount of water, a bit of lemon peel, fresh ginger, cinnamon and a few cloves, then boil until the fruit become soft. I leave it overnight for the spices to really impregnate the liquid and in the morning strain the liquid into another pot. These I heat again and add as much jam sugar (sugar with pectin) as will dissolve, then pour it into sterilised jam jars.

Hedgerow jelly is delicious with strong cheese or with pork sausages or roasts. At this time of the year, the medical herbalists of Botanica Medica are very busy helping people with colds and 'flu, and yet we almost never get ill; I feel quite sure this has something to do with the protection provided by hedgerow jelly.

Now is the time to remember that old saying "Many haws, many snaws." If your local hawthorn tree or hedge is groaning under the weight of haws this year, make a mental note to see if we have lots of snow this winter.

Hogweed – The Love Plant (*Heracleum sphondylium*)

Many people believe that hogweed is dangerous and can cause blisters. It is, in fact, the giant hogweed (*Heracleum mantegazzianum*) that causes the severe third degree burns; the native British, smaller common hogweed (*Heracleum sphondylium*) may cause less severe skin rashes.

Nonetheless, it would be advisable to take care around all hogweed plants. Having said that, it appears to be relished by foragers who make flower bud tempura, amongst other recipes.

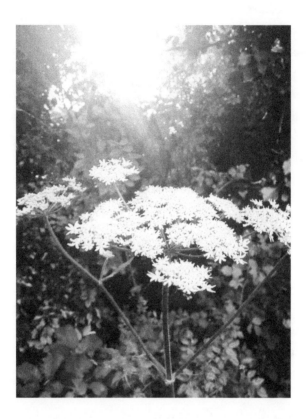

With blisters in mind, imagine my astonishment when I discovered that, in Romania, the common hogweed is celebrated as an aphrodisiac and stamina tonic. They call it the Love Plant, or Romanian Ginseng. The whole plant is known to be a powerful sexual tonic. By stimulating the activity of the ovaries and the testes, it raises hormone levels and the Romanians use the plant to treat impotence and infertility. Older folk use it as a rejuvenating herb for mental and physical fatigue and for premature menopause. It is said that women who have taken the herb to help them through the menopause suddenly find themselves pregnant again!

Although the plant is reputed to lower the blood pressure due to its general vaso-dilating effects, it specifically dilates the blood vessels of the genitals. It is a relaxing herb, acting as an antispasmodic to the uterine muscles as well as reducing anxiety. As such, I suppose, hogweed makes the perfect aphrodisiac.

However, I do not advocate its use as I have no personal experience of this plant nor could I find any scientific evidence for the above, although I have found plenty of Romanian herbal pharmacy websites selling the herbal tablets. Looking at the plant, we see that it is big and strong and very fertile, so perhaps it is telling us what it can be used for.

Angelica (*Angelica archangelica*) and Alexanders (*Angelica sylvestris*)

The splendid angelica stands tall and handsome, radiating the essence of strength and power. Legend tells us that it received its wonderful name, 'the archangel of angels', because the plant once saved an entire village from plague. With hundreds dying every day in nearby towns and villages of the dreaded disease, a village priest despaired for the safety of his parish and he prayed. The Archangel Michael came to him and instructed that he must give the people this plant. Each person held a piece of the root under his or her tongue and no-one died. So the plant was named in thanks to the angelic power of protection. Wisdom lies in old stories and they should not be dismissed too lightly… Science has found angelica to be powerfully antimicrobial, particularly against one of our modern day horrors, *Clostridium difficile*[22].

It has been widely used "against contagion for purifying the blood, and for curing every conceivable malady: as a sovereign remedy for poisons, agues and all infectious maladies." Angelica is particularly famous as a lung tonic, for general debility and for rheumatism. The plant tones the lungs and warms and strengthens the rest of the body. Indeed, in the olden days it was used against tuberculosis, pleurisy and pneumonia. This is a rather forgotten herb, but I love to use this plant for those whose lungs feel like they have closed up or who have developed coughs in the cold damp weather. The plant is powerfully antimicrobial, expectorant and a bronchial tonic, perfect for those weakened by lung infections and chesty coughs.

For Chest Infections

It is quite simple to make an infusion of the leaf with ginger, honey and lemon for a chest cold but, if you prefer, here is an older recipe: "Boil down gently for three hours a handful of angelica root in a quart of water and then strain it off and add liquid Narbonne honey or best virgin honey sufficient to make it into a balsam or syrup. Take two tablespoonsful every night and morning, as well as several times in the day." Do note the hearty doses required to rid yourself of nasty chest infections; a few drops here and there will do nothing to cure bronchitis.

More delectable pleasures have been attributed to this plant in the form of the popular aromatic herbal liqueurs distilled by European monks to aid digestion, giving us a clue to more of its many thera-peutic uses. The root and seeds have a warming, tonifying effect on the digestive system, reducing the indigestion and flatulence that so many people experience after eating heavy meals. Angelica is famous in all the old herbals for rheumatism and, whilst we do not use it for this purpose these days, this may be due to its warming actions.

Further, "The dryed roote made into pouder, and taken in wine or other drinke, will abate the rage of lust in young persons." Seems a shame to spoil the healthy lust of youth, but that was the rather monas-tic advice of the apothecary to King James I, Mr Parkinson, in 1629.

Older generations ate the plant as a vegetable by blanching the leaf stalks and eating them with bread and butter. In the days when sugar was a rare and costly treat, angelica was used to sweeten desserts such as stewed pears and rhubarb, and this would be delicious; but do be careful if you are diabetic because it can raise blood sugar levels. An alternative option would be to use sweet cicely seedpods, which have a sweet aniseed-like taste but do not raise blood sugars.

Scientists are discovering many of the marvellous properties of this plant, and a lot of the discoveries do not reflect the plant's traditional uses. Both the root and the seeds act significantly on the nervous system by calming anxiety and at the same time improving memory. Clinical trials testing angelica on dementia patients saw an improvement in symptoms such as delusions, agitation and anxiety[23] and it also significantly suppressed the duration of convulsions and improved the recovery of epileptic seizures in other clinical trials[24,25]. Another window of interest for scientists is that the seeds and root are able significantly to slow or halt the progression of pancreatic and breast cancers[26,27].

Wild angelica and garden angelica can be used interchangeably, but the garden variety is the stronger medicinally and can easily be grown in any cottage garden where it looks very statuesque.

Hops (*Humulus lupulus*)

Hops are often to be found tangled in the hedgerows as escapees from hops fields, now long gone. For the herbalist, hops offer many opportunities for rebalancing and comforting our patients.

Hops, as we all know, are used to flavour beers, but the men who drink beer in large quantities are usually unaware that this herb acts as an anaphrodisiac, hence brewer's droop. This quencher of the male libido can be used temporarily to cool a man's ardour if his partner cannot match his bedtime stamina. It achieves this because hops are rich in phyto-oestrogens (plant oestrogens), so it is also used in products that promise to enhance the female bust.

Herbalists are not often asked to achieve either of these effects for our patients, so we tend to use the phyto-oestrogens instead to cool the hot flushes of menopausal women. This herb is absolutely perfect for women who have reached the age when their oestrogen levels start to decline, with their sleep badly disrupted by hot flushes and drenching sweats. Very many women find that they are woken every few hours, so burning with heat and soaked in perspiration that they need to change their bedclothes and stand at the window to cool down. By the time the flush has passed, however, they are wide awake and can't fall asleep again. It is very debilitating.

Hops not only supplements the declining oestrogens, it is also a hypnotic herb. This means it deeply relaxes the mind and promotes sleep. So this herb does a marvellous double job of reducing the flushes to barely any, and if a lady does wake in the night she will drop off to sleep again very easily. Hops can be combined very nicely with some sage from the garden and a few flowers of red clover to provide a very effective menopause tea.

Hops offer another wonderful service to the modern human in the form of relaxing the gut. I see so many patients suffering with irritable bowel syndrome and one of the main causes is the stress and agitation of modern life. When we rush about in a state of unacknowledged but constant angst, we are locked into the sympathetic nervous system state. This means that while we are constantly ready for fight-and-flight, our digestive enzymes have been shut off and the blood is diverted to our muscles and brain so that we can cope with the state of emergency that our body believes us to be in.

There is a lot to be said for the time when good manners urged us to sit down and eat in a convivial atmosphere. Without sufficient digestive enzymes, our food cannot be broken down and absorbed;

instead it remains undigested and in that warm moist environment begins to ferment, producing very uncomfortable gas. Our sympathetic nervous state also encourages the involuntary muscles in our intestines to clench up, and the normal smooth peristaltic movement is interrupted by uncoordinated spasms.

When we drink a cup of hops tea or some tincture, we immediately notice the bitterness. Although unpleasant to taste, our stomachs recognise the bitterness as a signal to secrete digestive enzymes. In the meantime, the liquid quickly slips into the bloodstream and is taken to the brain, which is calmed and sends messages back to the gut that it too can relax. The muscles unclench, digestive enzymes flow, the person relaxes and irritable bowel symptoms melt away.

If you can find some hops, you will notice that in early September the prettiest little cones have formed. Once they have reached full size, we can harvest them. If you have a spare pillowcase, do fill it with hops cones and lavender flowers and use this as a sleeping pillow if you have trouble with insomnia. Some people like to include wormwood sprigs to enhance their dreams.

Irritable Bowel Syndrome Tea

1 cone of hops flowers
1 teaspoon of fennel seeds
3 slices of fresh ginger
1 chamomile teabag

Comfrey, Knitbone (*Symphytum officinalis*)

The many names of this herb say it all: knitbone, knitback, bruisewort, boneset and consolida. Its botanical name is derived from the Greek word 'symphyto' meaning to unite. This plant has the ability to stimulate the regrowth of bone tissue, yet not only this but all connective tissue, from which our entire body is made up. Therefore we value this plant for the repairing of all wounds, breaks, ulcers, erosions, cuts, surgery and so on.

The wound healing action is so powerful that, as student herbalists, we were urged to be certain that the wound is thoroughly cleaned before applying comfrey as it will heal over the dirt, sealing it in. It is a wonderful herb but should be used with care.

Caution: Most important, if you are going to wild harvest, is to make absolutely certain that you are harvesting comfrey and not foxglove (see the photograph of foxglove in July), which has chemicals that can affect the heart.

Secondly, you need to make sure that you use the correct species, which is the common comfrey and not the rough comfrey or the Russian comfrey. The best idea would be to buy the plant from a reputable herb grower or to buy the herb from a medical herbalist. The official comfrey described above is distinguished from Russian and rough comfrey by a leaf wing that runs down the leaf stalk right to the stem; the rough and Russian comfrey leaves do not run like wings down the leaf stalk to the stem.

Thirdly, it is best only to use the leaf internally and for a maximum period of six weeks. The root can be used externally quite safely.

If you were to cut the root of comfrey, you will discover a slimy exudate much like marshmallow. This slime, which we call mucilage, gives the same protective effect on raw mucus membranes and skin tissue as marshmallow, but it offers something extra being rich in allantoin, which stimulates the proliferation and repair of cells. On the skin, the effect is very similar to snail slime, which cosmetics laboratories are using in their beauty creams – can you believe it? The slime is reported to heal and repair red inflamed skin and to lock in moisture. Personally it does not appeal to me to use the slime of imprisoned snails on my face, when comfrey provides the same action abundantly.

However Mary Beith, author of Healing Threads (Birlinn Ltd, 2004), argues that harvesting snail slime is not cruel and thus there really is no need to incur the wrath of the Gastropods' Rights lobby! Much as snails in my garden drive me mad, I would still vote for their freedoms and rights. As an aside, she mentions that in the past Scottish people used to chop snails up fine and hang them in flannel bags in front of the fire. Their oily drippings were captured and used for rheumatism, tuberculosis or whooping cough; a more disgusting remedy I cannot imagine.

Back to the mucilage of comfrey, which is thick, slimy and soothing to bleeding stomach ulcers, and ulcerated intestines. The herb protects and stimulates the healing of these damaged tissues, but it is most important that the underlying cause of these conditions be addressed. The leaf or root can be used on varicose ulcers, which refuse to heal, or slow to heal surgical wounds, but of course, its most famous use is to promote the healing of broken bones.

Vegetarian 'Fried Fish'

Collect some leaves of the correct common comfrey, rinse and dry them. Now dip the leaves into whisked egg and then into self-raising flour. Drop the leaves into hot oil in a frying pan and fry them gently until golden. Take them out and blot off the excess oil with kitchen towel then serve them with a squeeze of lemon juice and a fresh rocket and Parmesan salad. This is a most delicious dish.

Valerian (*Valeriana officinalis*)

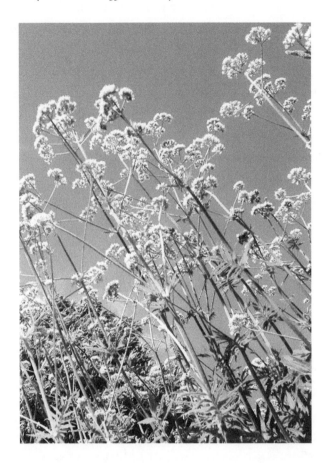

The pungent scent of valerian is said to be so attractive to rats that it was used in rat traps, and Mrs Grieves suggests that, "The famous Pied Piper of Hamlin owed his irresistible power over rats to the fact that he secreted valerian roots about his person."

Well, certainly the effect on cats is that they become quite ecstatic and amorous. In fact, I once came home to find my neighbour's very large Norwegian Forest cat lying upside-down in my herb basket with his head hanging over a bag of valerian. He had a look of joyous rapture on his face.

The ecstatic amorous effect does not extend to humans, alas, or I would be a very wealthy lady by now. Acting on the human being, valerian is deeply calming, helping our over-busy minds to see the wood for the trees. Very often I have patients who are terribly upset about something and this herb helps them to gain a little psychological distance and some perspective, so that they can think clearly. The herb quietens the mind, allowing the agitated person to drop off to sleep where their energies can be restored. In contrast to chemical drugs, valerian allows a deep and restful sleep, but one wakes fully alert and ready for the day. It also calms the mind but does not dull it, so it is quite possible to give a business presentation with calmness and clarity.

Life wasn't always so frenetic. My old herbal medicine teacher told me that in the 19th century people were "bored to shrieks", but now we are a generation of stressed out mentally exhausted heaps. It is interesting to note that herbs are used for different purposes in different lands, or at different times. In past centuries, valerian was principally used for hysteria, hypochondria, epilepsy, persistent irritable coughs, neuralgia or infected wounds. Earlier in the 16th century it was used as a 'counter poison.'

One of the old names of valerian is 'phu', onomatopoeically describing its effects on the nasals. The patients in our clinic often complain about the pungent smell of old socks when we work with valerian; in fact, an irate woman once asked, "What is that dreadful smell that seeps out from under your door and reeks the street?" What could I say, other than I am rather fond of its smell. To me, it has quite an animal smell to it. Nonetheless, she would have been amazed to learn that in the medieval ages it was actually used as a culinary spice and as a perfume! The Anglo-Saxons used the plant as a salad and the Scots considered that a broth was worthless if it did not contain valerian. I have to say that it is probably the herb I value most in our apothecaries.

October

Autumn is such a magical season in the hedgerows and fields. Everything seems to be floating gently downwards, back to the earth. Early morning mists hover over the fields, droplets clinging to glittering spider webs. The sun lies low in the sky and falling birch leaves flash like golden coins, leaving deep beds of mulch. Female deer nervously nibble beneath towering chestnut trees whilst rival stags bellow their primal challenge at each other, as they have done for thousands and thousands of years.

At this misty time of the year, it is quite common when walking across manure-rich fields where cows have spent the summer, to come across rings of mushrooms. In the past, it was thought that faeries danced in these rings at night, sometimes with a glowworm for a lamp

and a grasshoppers for musicians, so they were called faery rings or
faery dances. An account of what befell a certain gentleman, whilst
walking one evening, might serve as a warning to those of us who like
to roam the fields after sunset:

"In the year 1633-4, soon after I had entered into my grammar at the
Latin School at Yatton Keynel, our curate Mr. Hart was annoyd one
night by these elves or fayries comming over the downes. It being near
darke, and approaching one of the faery dances as the common people
call them in these parts, he all at once sawe an innumerable quantitie
of pygmies or very small people dancing rounde and rounde, and
singing and making all maner of small noyses. So being very greatly
amaz'd and yet not being able, as he says, to run away from them, being
as he supposes kepte there in a kinde of enchantment. They no sooner
perceave him but they surrounde him on all sides, and what betwixt
feare and amazement, he fell downe scarecely knowing what he did;
and thereupon these little creatures pinch'd him all over and made a

sorte of quick humming noyse all the time; but at length they left him, and when the sun rose he found himself exactly in the midst of one these faery dances. This relation I had from him myselfe a few dayes after he was so tormented; but when I and my bedfellow Stump wente soon afterwards at night time to the dances on the downes, we sawe none of the elves or fayries. But indeed it is saide they seldom appeare to any persons who go to seeke for them." (John Aubrey, recounted in John Ramsbottom, Mushrooms and Toadstools, Collins 1953)

Horseradish (*Armoracia rusticana*)

A hearty herb, which 17th century herbalist John Parkinson rather snobbishly refers to as being an appropriate sauce for "strong labour-ing men in Germany and England, but not for tender and gentle stomaches." Perhaps we have become more vulgar, for horseradish sauce is not only a popular condiment now but also an excellent medicine for our cold winters.

The pungency is due to a mustard oil called allyl isothiocyanate, which is released on crushing, and it is the heat of this mustard oil for which we value horseradish. The root is also rich in vitamin C. Essentially the root, when used as a medicine, is a circulatory stimu-lant bringing warmth where needed; it is also an excellent expectorant and broncho-dilator. The root is rich in sulphur, which attracts and binds deep cellular toxins, eliminating them from the body. In this way the herb kills infection and stimulates the elimination of waste products. Being a circulatory stimulant, horseradish dilates the blood vessels and, in doing so, flushes the tissues with fresh cleansed blood. It also encourages the kidneys to move the waste products from the blood into the urine for elimination.

Horseradish has a particular affinity for the respiratory system. I make a horseradish tincture or syrup to use for deep phlegmy coughs, which are associated with a person feeling chilled. The horseradish warms the bronchi by dilating the capillaries, loosening and expectorating tough phlegm so that the lungs feel relieved of their heaviness. The mustard oil kills the bacteria lurking in green mucus. It is very helpful for those who are chilly, with wheezy, deep, infected coughs and rather severe viral or bacterial infections. The herb would be just as useful for congested sinuses; by opening the blood vessels, the solid mucus is diluted and suddenly the clogged up sinuses start streaming. I think of it as bringing back to life the nearly dead…

We live in times when hurry and worry can permeate many people's every moment. Stress of this type stimulates the sympathetic nervous system and shuts off the secretion of digestive enzymes. Most people are unaware of this process. As we get older, our stomach becomes 'cold'. We have an overall feeling of chilliness and our digestive juice is less effective. When this happens, it feels like the food remains undigested for hours, with burping, fermentation and flatulence. Horseradish warms the stomach and its pungency stimulates the flow of digestive enzymes allowing the food to be broken down and absorbed.

It is worth noting John Parkinson's advice above that it is not an appropriate herb for those with tender stomachs such as you would have if you suffer from gastritis, stomach ulcers, or any inflammation of the digestive system. However, if you deem yourself to have a strong rustic stomach, this is my favourite horseradish recipe.

Fresh Horseradish Sauce

Fresh horseradish root peeled and finely grated
½ cup of double cream
½ cup of plain Greek yoghurt

Blend the cream and the yoghurt and then stir in as much horseradish as you can into the creamy blend. Dollop generously onto a steak or into baby jacket potatoes, topped with a small piece of smoked salmon.

A Chest Cough Syrup

Fresh horseradish root peeled and grated
½ cup of vegetable glycerine or honey

Push as much grated horseradish as you can into the glycerine or honey and soak for a day, then strain it; keep it for no longer that a month, in a glass bottle in the fridge.
To use, take one teaspoon three or four times a day after food to ease congested lungs or sinuses.

Horse Chestnut (*Aesculus hippocastanum*)

In the 1600s, Mr Nicolas Culpeper liked to that say, "Any boy who can eat an egg knows this plant", and 'conkers' is still a popular game with children. The beautiful horse chestnut tree was so named because the nuts were considered unfit for human consumption; indeed, within the seed lie saponins, which can irritate the stomach if eaten in large quantities.

These fat seeds were used to feed horses and cattle in Europe, but it was necessary to leach the nut in water overnight and then throw the water away before grinding the seeds to a meal, which was fed to the animals. During World War I, animals were fed in this manner so that the grain could be saved for human consumption. So, indirectly, the horse chestnuts did feed humans during those brave years.

These days, medical herbalists use the seed for their tonic effect on veins and arteries. It is superb in its ability to help those suffering with bleeding piles, bleeding gums, varicose veins and swollen ankles. A very pretty young woman came to see me one day suffering with anxiety about going to Ascot. She worried that because she would have to stand all day, her legs would swell, causing her great discomfort. She came to see me only two weeks before the event, which is not a lot of time for herbs to do their job; but after the event, she reported that although it was an extremely hot day her legs had been absolutely fine.

People tell me that they leave conkers on their windowsills as they keep spiders away. But the ancient people respected Grandmother Spider who weaves the web of life, and I too like spiders.

Sweet Chestnut (*Castanea sativa*)

The sweet chestnut is another enormous tree whose nuts are equally relished by deer, squirrels and humans. There is a lovely old saying that, "Chestnuts are a delicacy for princes and a lusty food for rustic youths." Now this is interesting because if you ever want to find the deer during the rutting season, you shall find them beneath the chestnut trees; and during the summer the flowers emit the smell of sperm. That said, they do not have any reputation as an aphrodisiac but rather as a treatment for coughing. Old recipes suggest crushing the chestnuts with honey, then taking teaspoons of this lovely concoction to soothe paroxysmal coughs such as whooping cough.

Monk's Hood (*Aconitum napellus*)

Now, amongst all these wonderful characters of the hedgerows, there has to be a villain! The undisputed femme fatale of the hedgerow must be the stunningly beautiful and utterly deadly aconite. How alluring she is, with tall willowy stems and deep purple delphinium-like flowers, and one is irresistibly drawn closer to look and possibly even pick a flower. But graceful beauty belies her baneful nature.

Caution: The innocent, picking a stem, is likely to become severely poisoned if the sap simply enters a small wound. The symptoms include convulsions, turning purple in the face, and severe body pains or suffocation.

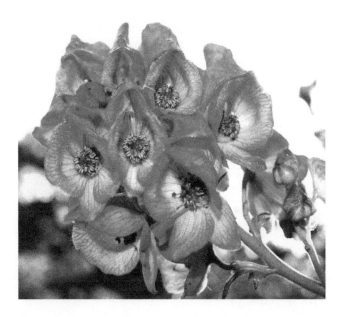

This plant is rich in an alkaloid called aconitine, known as the Queen of Poisons. Death comes quickly and coldly: the nerve messages are blocked, circulation and respiration are shut down, and all the while there is a sensation of ants crawling over the skin. There is no antidote. A gardener (only) once dug up and cooked aconite bulbs with his Jerusalem artichokes and, within three hours, he and his friend were dead. Well, a gardener of all people should know better than to plant a deadly poisonous plant in his kitchen garden.

Aconite is also known as wolfbane. Arrows were dipped into the poison for hunting wolves, bears and panthers, and the plant was also mixed into meat and left out to kill wolves. However, as the saying goes, the difference between a medicine and a poison is the dose, and aconite can be used as a powerfully painkilling liniment externally for neuralgia and rheumatic pain. But I have never had the courage to use it.

Airmid's Cloak

Like all healers, medical herbalists dearly wish that we could heal all of our patients perfectly, but we are human and this is not realistic. We do, however, manage to heal most people who come to see us although the following story tells why we might not always be successful.

Long, long ago, at a time when the gods still walked the Earth, there lived one called Dian Cecht. He was the god of healing and renowned as the most powerful healer in the land but he had a fierce temper. The Tuatha de Danaan of the faery race was ruled by King Nuada, who lost his hand in a battle. For the king to rule, he had to be perfect, so Dian Cecht fashioned for him a silver hand that could move like a living hand. But Dian Cecht had a son called Miach who had superseded his father's skills in healing. He created for the king an arm out of flesh and blood, making the king perfect again and able to rule.

Dian Cecht had the fury of a god when he discovered that his son was a better healer than him, and in his rage he approached his son, raised his sword and smote him a blow across the neck. Miach looked at his father and then drew his hand across the wound, completely healing it. The father, incensed by this insolence struck him a blow across his head with the sword, cutting deeply into the skull. Again Miach healed the wound instantly. So Dian Cecht, in his jealous rage, raised his sword again and with a crashing blow cut off his son's head. This wound could not be healed and the young god died in his weeping father's arms and was buried.

Through the winter the grave lay bare and his sister Airmid visited it regularly. It was in the springtime that she noticed green shoots appearing over the grave in the shape of her brother's body. Then she noticed that chamomile was growing over his stomach, betony over his head and lungwort over his chest; she realised that Miach was trying to teach her the herbs of the fields so that his healing skills would not be lost. Carefully Airmid collected the herbs and spread them out on her cloak according to his shape, so that she would remember for which body part each herb was to be used.

But on this day, Dian Cecht came also to visit his son's grave and erupted in fury as he immediately recognised what Airmid was doing. He seized the cloak and shook it violently, scattering the herbs. Airmid, the goddess of herbal healing, remembered most of the herbs and their uses, but some say that this is why a herbalist cannot cure every ill: some of that great knowledge was lost to the winds at the whim of a jealous god.

Samhain

The ghouls and skeletons of Hallowe'en parties recall a much older tradition where our Celtic ancestors celebrated death and renewal as part of the cycle of life. The same goes for trick-or-treating, which reflects the trickster time of year when people would play pranks on their neighbours, like hiding horses in different fields.

Today, the ancient festival is still celebrated as Samhain (pronounced Sow-een) beginning on the eve of the 31st of October until the 1st of November. This is a time when it is said that the veil between this world and the spirit world is at its thinnest, so it is a time to contact those who have passed over. This is a sacred time of the year when we honour the ancestors who have gone before us, remembering them and thanking them for their efforts that enabled us to live our lives as we do. We honour the old and wise traditions and can also use this time to let go of anything that no longer serves us in our lives. Without the death of the old, the birth of the new cannot happen; so we look back on the past before looking forward to the future.

To celebrate Samhain you might like to make bread in the traditional manner and place little charms or folded notes within it, giving thanks for what is past and making wishes for what you would like to bring into your life.

November

As the hedgerow cycle slips slowly away from the warmth of summer, the cold mists rise wraith-like off the rivers and lakes to act like an anaesthetic. As they drift over the plants, the coldness penetrates into the tissues, causing their vital forces to sink narcotically into the safety of the deep, dark earth. Here the nutrients gathered during the warmth of summer are stored in the roots to provide nourishment for the plant and animals of the fields during the winter. It is a time when we too can sink deeply into our own psyche to find the quietness of our souls and to search around our inner underworld to find our own roots, understanding and inspiration, and to rest within Mother Earth.

Elecampane (*Inula helenium*)

The roots are now swollen with the starch and stored nutrients of summer, sufficient to nourish the plant through the winter, so this is the time when herbalists harvest root herbs such as elecampane. Lifting this root is a wonderfully aromatic experience. The thick roots should be followed with muddy fingers and gently pulled from the earth, then snip off these thick finger-like protrusions and replant the root ball. Once the roots have been harvested, they are scrubbed clean and carefully sliced to allow them to dry before turning them into one of our most valuable tinctures for winter.

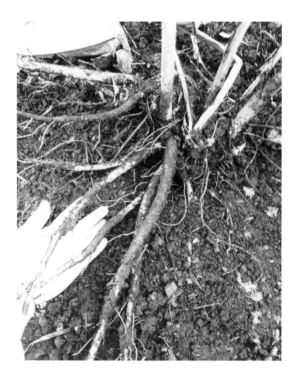

At this cold and damp time of year, we use Inula for chest infections, when the mucus is difficult to expectorate or when it has become greeny-yellow with infection. The pungent warmth of the roots loosens the thick, sticky catarrh so that it may be more easily coughed up; but at the same time, it helps to disinfect the lungs. I love to combine elecampane with angelica and horseradish for chest infections.

Nature is very complete in her medicinal gifts, and elecampane offers a perfect example. An action that is largely forgotten about Inula is that it is a vermifuge – it kills intestinal worms and opportunistic, unfriendly gut bacteria. If a patient suffers from dysbiosis (too much unfriendly bacteria in the gut), the herbalist's approach would be to kill the unfriendly gut residents and then boost the friendly bacteria population with probiotics; the probiotics are also fed with prebiotics. A common prebiotic food is inulin, which we find in abundance within the root of Inula. We also must remember that the roots bring up a type of probiotic called 'soil borne organisms' from the earth. So now, with one plant, we kill the pathogenic bacteria of the gut, which can cause irritable bowel syndrome or inflammatory bowel disease. At the same time, probiotics in the form of soil borne organisms are provided, along with the prebiotic food to sustain their growth.

The Yew Tree (*Taxus baccata*)

The fact that yew trees are often found in graveyards, are extremely poisonous and have almost black-green foliage, has popularly contributed to their association with death. Legends don't help its dark reputation when they tell us that the nightmare sleeps in the tree on a nest of poets' bones. But let us get to know this venerable tree a little better, as plants have a much longer history than humans, and tucked away in their histories are wonderful secrets.

Yew is almost certainly the most ancient of our trees. The odd stray can be found in the hedgerows, but more often than not we find this grand tree in old churchyards; there are also still a very few ancient yew forests remaining in Britain such as at Kingley Vale in

West Sussex. It is known that the Druids revered this tree, probably because they are practically immortal, this representing the immorality of the soul. Ancient Druids believed in reincarnation and that the soul passes from one body to the next.

When the trunk becomes very old, it hollows out and the old branches sag to touch the earth where they take root and become new trees, albeit still attached to the old mother tree. In this way, one tree can spread, faery-ring-like, to form a grove of yew trees, and there is no reason why this should not continue forever if left undisturbed. The wood is extremely hard, resistant to water damage and very hard wearing. In 1911, a spear made from yew wood was excavated in Essex and dated to be around 450,000 years old.

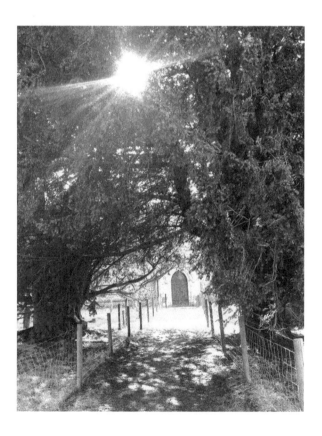

It is very difficult to measure the age of yews as the trunks hollow with age and the wood does not form tree rings. Until recently they were thought to be younger than botanists are currently suggesting, and there are many single trees still living in the British Isles that were previously estimated to be between 2,000 to 4,000 years old; but now they have been aged closer to 6,000 or 8,000 years old. At the time of Jesus they were over 4,000 years old. These trees were already 3,000 years old when Stonehenge was built and when the pharaohs ruled ancient Egypt. Still they live, like immortal gods to life. Extending even further back, *Taxus grandis*, which is almost indistinguishable from the modern *Taxus baccata*, is 140 million years old... these trees lived with the dinosaurs!

It is hard for us to imagine these vast tracts of time as being part of the lifespan of a single tree. Perhaps it is easier to link it to a well-known reference point in our history, such as the signing of the Magna Carta that took place under a yew tree 800 years ago on the island of Ankerwyke, surrounded by the water meadows of Runnymede. The site was chosen because the wide open fields made ambush from either side impossible and Ankerwyke was the home of an established convent, the ruins of which are still to be seen; thus desecration of the sanctity of the island would not have made good publicity.

During the Saxon era, Runnymede was known as Rune-mede or the 'meadow of the runes'. On the island of Ankerwyke stands a very old yew, now thought to be at least 2,500 years old, so at the time of signing Magna Carta it would have been well over 1,700 years old. Historians believe that this was one of the trees under which the Druids, who were the pre-Roman judges and law-givers, gave council. We may propose that the Druids had been using this spot for several hundreds of years before the Romans came, as the tree would have been about 600 years old at the time of the Romans. The runes were imported to Britain with the Saxons around 500 AD and, judging from the name Rune-mede, it is possible that they were read for a significant period of time by village shamanic figures under this yew. So we can suggest that the Ankerwyke yew provided the significant place under which council could be held for the Druids who venerated yews, for the Anglo-Saxons and later for King John and the barons, as a place traditionally associated with wise council and law-making.

But why, we might ask, are yews associated with church grave-yards? Clearly, some yews are much older than the church building itself. Many churches were built directly atop ancient sacred sites such as burial mounds. When Pope Gregory wrote to Augustine in Britain in the year 594 AD, he advised him, "…not to destroy pagan temples, but rather to replace the idols with the relics of saints, to sprinkle the old precincts with holy water and rededicate them, because people come more readily to the places where they have been accustomed to pray…" Christianity simply absorbed the old religion and its places, so that the old gods and goddesses morphed into saints, sacred springs became holy wells, and the sacred places where people used to worship the pagan gods became churches with the revered old trees still in situ.

The ancient people of Britain didn't seem to see the dead as dead-and-gone but rather inhabiting another realm. The dead were still alive and available to them and it is known that the Druids were perfectly happy to leave a debt unpaid, since it could be repaid in the afterlife.

The ancestors could be accessed if people went to certain places at certain times of the year; Samhain, for instance, would be a time-por-tal. The people may have gone to the burial mounds to communicate with those who had passed to the otherworld with the intention of gaining advice, inspiration or to honour them. We can only guess.

For the people of ancient Britain, the entire landscape was sacred. It is my personal belief that the islands of Britain were themselves a giant altar where the people moved in a semi-continuous pilgrimage from sacred points in the landscape to burial mounds and standing stone temples in order to honour their deities and the spirits of the land. Springs, mountains, trees and burial mounds all formed part of the sacred landscape.

Many of these burial mounds are over 5,000 years old and it has been noted that yews of over 4,000 years old seem to have been planted on the north side of the burial mounds. The Celts planted yews on an east-west line through the centre of the burial mound, and later the Saxons planted yews on the south side. Some suggest that the yew houses the souls of the dead who cannot find their way home. Perhaps the tree provides a safe haven for lost souls and perhaps thousands of years ago the people considered that they could communicate with the dead through the living spirit of the yew because trees were seen to be in touch with the underworld by their roots, with the upper world by branches in the sky, and with Middle Earth, our mortal plane of existence. We don't really know with any certainty what the yew meant to the people who planted them, but we do know that the tree was sacred, it was planted consciously on sacred sites, particularly burial sites, and that these sites often became church sites in during the Christian period.

Some modern authors suggest that the yew is a manifestation of a god or, if you feel more comfortable, that it might have been thought of as a god. Looking at the common roots of old languages we find a fascinating correlation. In Old English yew is called 'iw' or 'eow' or 'eoh'. In Middle Dutch and Low German it was called 'iewe' or 'uwe'. The Celts named it 'yewar' and the Early Modern English called it 'yewe'. All these words may have been pronounced 'yeo-weh', which is very close to the Hebrew pronouncement of Jahevahe or YHVH, the tetragrammaton for the sacred, therefore unpronounceable, name of God.

Caution: The association with life and death continues still into very recent times. The tree is so toxic that the leaves were used to poison arrow tips.

Yet this very poison has been found to save life too. The Pacific yew *Taxus brevifolia* provides the drug Taxol, which is a chemotherapeutic drug used to fight breast, ovarian and some lung cancers, and it appears to be successful too. Even though the tree is associated with graveyards and poisons, it seems the old Druids were onto something when they revered it as a tree of life and death.

But now there is a sorry twist in this lovely tale. I once attended a lecture on the subject of 'The Green Wood and Yews' by Professor Ronald Hutton, Professor of History at the University of Bristol. Ronald has a way of being highly entertaining as he completely debunks all our knowledge by thorough historical research. He explained that yews are probably not as old as we think they are and that it is likely that the Christians adopted them in their churchyards because they were the only trees that the Druids had not tarnished with their pagan beliefs.

Now, on a lighter note, a legend tells us that when the world was young the yew tree longed to look bright and beautiful, so the faeries gave it leaves of gold. Yew was so happy with her golden cloak but robbers came along and stripped her. So the faeries consoled her with leaves of scintillating crystal but a hailstorm passed and all the crystal was shattered. This time the faeries gifted yew with soft bright green leaves but animals ate the tender foliage. After this, the yew preferred the peace and solace of her dark foliage.

But all is not quite as it seems at first sight. Some years ago, I was sitting under a yew tree in an ancient graveyard reflecting on its associations with darkness and death, when a flash of light caught my eye. Rain had fallen not long before and the clouds had parted, allowing a ray of sunlight to pierce the raindrops clinging to the leaflets, so that each raindrop acted as a crystal prism; for a few minutes the tree was ablaze with thousands of shimmering jewels of red, orange, yellow, green, blue and violet. The sun moved behind the clouds again, but the yew had had her moment of crystalline glory, for light shines so much brighter against dark foliage.

Over the centuries, children have been attracted to the bright red, sweet fruit, this being the only part of the tree that is not poisonous. This sweet slimy fruit was relished and called snotty-gobbles or red snot, but I doubt that children would be allowed to eat its fruit these days!

Fly Agaric (*Amanita muscaria*)

November being the month when we have an abundance of mushrooms popping up in our fields and forests, I would like to tell a tale about the *Amanita muscaria* mushroom, which grows for about three weeks beneath the birch trees in November.

Amanita muscaria is the classic red and white, spotty fly agaric toadstool that features in Alice in Wonderland. Remember that Alice went down the rabbit hole, entering a strange underworld where relative to other objects she became either giant or tiny? An account from 1762 tells how American Indian shamans used to eat the mushroom to facilitate entering trance. During this state, the senses would become altered so that objects appeared to be either very large or very small. When the shaman used plants to enter the trance state, it was always with the sacred intention of entering the Underworld or the Upperworld to communicate with their gods. The mushroom was never indulged for recreational purposes but taken with great reverence. Shamanic practices the world over are remarkably similar and, as the American Indians used the mushroom to induce trance, so too did the Siberian shaman.

There are many suggestions concerning the origins of the Father Christmas story, and this is only one that may or may not hold any truth at all. Nevertheless, it is a nice fireside story...

It is possible that the story of Father Christmas is a sanitised retelling of an earlier Siberian shamanic practice. After feeding his reindeer

Amanita mushroom, the shaman would capture the urine from the reindeer and drink it. In doing so, many of the constituents that cause negative side effects were filtered through the reindeer's liver, but the psychotropic effects were still available to the shaman and facilitated his trance entry into the spirit world. He had no sense of time as he met with and learned from his spirit guides, and when he was done he would come out of trance bringing to his people the gifts of spiritual wisdom.

Looking at our image of Father Christmas, we see a venerable old man (the shaman) dressed in a red suit, lined with white fur (the colours of the mushroom), flying through the air (in trance to the Upperworlds), carried by his troop of reindeer (whose urine furnished the 'trip'), distributing gifts (of wisdom) to the whole wide world in a single night (as if time were elastic).

It is important to point out that medical herbalists never use *Amanita muscaria* as a medicine, nor are shamanic practices part of our therapy. But still, it is interesting to look a little closer into our past and into the practices of herbalists from other cultures using the same plants that we find in our hedgerows.

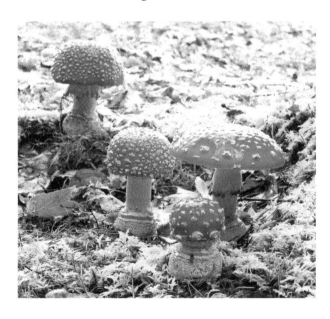

December

Yule, the Winter Solstice

For three days around the 21st of December, time seems to stand still. During these days, the hours of darkness are at their longest in the year and then, very slowly at first, the sun grows in strength and daylight hours begin to lengthen. To the ancients, the winter solstice was hugely important as the time when the Sun King is reborn. Light and warmth return to the land. To celebrate, mistletoe is cut as a symbol of the masculine and the sign of light. Squashing a mistletoe berry, we notice that it has the consistency of sperm. It is sometimes called 'the sperm of the gods', and the luminescent colour reflects the weak and pale sun. Bright berries of holly, mistletoe, candles and shining trinkets all reflect the returning of light.

Although the sun grows stronger with each passing day, the days are still dark and winter is at its harshest between now and Imbolc. The energy of the trees is nestling deep within the earth, as are the pregnant foxes and hedgehogs and seeds. Life is incubating deep inside Mother Earth. There is not much to do in the hedgerow or the garden at this time of the year, but we too can make plans and incubate ideas. So we follow the trees and allow our focus to sink deeply into the core of our being, resting during the dark months and drawing from nature, so that we may emerge renewed in the springtime. This is the time of reflection and potential.

Holly (*Ilex aquifolium*)

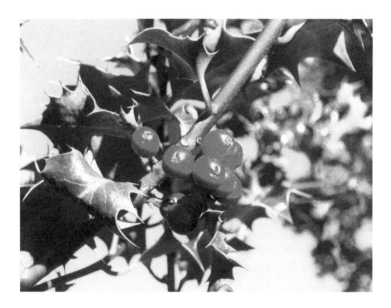

Holly is a plant of protection, a tree that acts as a guardian. Pliny informs us that planting holly near the house protects the home from poisons, lightning and witchcraft. Romans gave holly wreaths to brides to protect the couple from evil. The strong thick growth of the tree trimmed into a hedge makes an impenetrable barrier, guarding our homes and protecting against those who may feel jealous, perhaps coveting our possessions and, of course, Dr Bach prescribed holly for feelings of jealousy and envy. Druids use the holly to reinforce the masculine energies of strength, protection and defence, unconditional love and wisdom: to fight the just cause, if necessary.

According to folklore, holly should never be cut down and there is the inevitable story of a farmer who wanted a holly tree cut down but his labourers absolutely refused to do the deed. So the farmer found someone else who did not believe in these old wives' tales and, rather predictably, the man was dead within three months of cutting the tree.

Two thousand years ago, the Romans celebrated Saturnalia from the 17th to the 23rd of December and during this time they decorated their homes with holly. The Celts hung it in their roundhouses as a home to the Sylvan spirits, the spirits of the grove. During the dark days of winter, the shining leaves and bright red berries stand out as a beacon of light against the dark. This tree is a symbol of the winter solstice, which celebrates the rebirth of the Mabon, the child Sun King. From this time onwards, the sun grows in strength again.

It is noted that rabbits love to eat the bark of the tree, and when a stick is given to domestic rabbits it will act as a tonic, restoring their appetite. As medical herbalists we do not use the plant, but the folk of older times were made of much sterner stuff; throughout England, holly thrashing was used to treat chilblains, arthritis and a stiff neck. We don't do that to our patients anymore!

Mistletoe (*Viscum album*)

Mistletoe grows as a parasitic plant on apple and oak trees, amongst others, and it is in winter when the branches are exposed that the balls of green growth are particularly visible, high up at the tops of the trees. The seed is usually stuck onto a tree by a bird; as a 16th century herbalist rather charmingly informs us, "The thrush shitith forth the mistleberry onto the tree." The seeds stick to the branches and begin to invade and grow. The plant grows by feeding parasitically off its host, like a cancer, and it is as a cancer treatment for which it is so well known.

Here, The Doctrine of Signatures once again shows us the interesting correlation, but there also are many scientific studies that attest to *Viscum album*'s ability to fight cancer using a number of mechanisms. Cancer, like mistletoe, feeds off its host, and it needs to take as much nutrition as needed from the host to fuel its greedy growth. A tumour does this by producing its own blood vessel system, known as angiogenesis, and mistletoe actually inhibits angiogenesis. The plant inhibits the growth of the blood vessels, thereby starving the tumour of the nutrition necessary for growth.

Unlike healthy cells, cancer cells do not die. As a medicine, mistletoe induces natural cell death, known as apoptosis, and in doing so kills cancer cells. Cancer has a strong link with inflammation, but mistletoe has specific anti-inflammatory actions that help to inhibit cancer cell growth.

Finally, we all have rogue cancer cells in our bloodstream every single day, which our immune system quickly snaps up so that they cannot grow into tumours. Mistletoe stimulates the natural killer cells within the immune system and these immune cells are directly involved in killing cancer cells.

Mistletoe also has another fascinating weapon against cancer in that it traps the chemotherapeutic drugs within the cancer cells by interrupting the malignant cells' detoxifying pump system. One clinical trial shows that mistletoe therapy significantly improved quality of life in the twenty-five people studied[28]. Another study concluded that mistletoe does not interact negatively with chemotherapy, and at higher doses enhances the killing of cancer cells[29]. In a third clinical trial the prevention of any recurrence of the tumour and the regression of the cancer was noted in 85% of the patients who used a mistletoe/chemotherapy combination. This particular study notes that pre-clinical and clinical trials have demonstrated tumour growth inhibition, stimulation of the immune system and improvement of the quality of life as known benefits of mistletoe therapy[30].

Medical herbalists also use *Viscum album* to help control high blood pressure and for many years have found this to be safe and effective. Modern scientific studies agree that mistletoe does reduce the blood pressure[31,32]. The herb dilates the arteries and slows the heartbeat to a more normal rhythm. So we find that we have reason to respect mistletoe for having a significant part to play in our two biggest modern killers, cancer and cardiac disease.

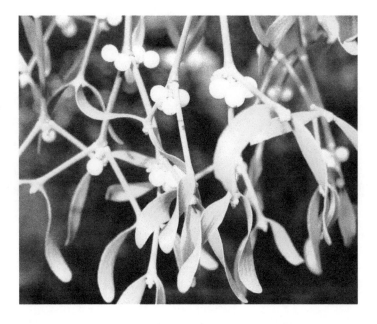

Certainly in ancient times mistletoe was a deeply respected plant and it was the most sacred plant of the Druids, possibly because it lived in the air between Heaven and Earth and never touched the soil. When they cut it during their sacred ceremonies, it was caught before it landed on the soil, thus preserving its heavenly energies. The ancient people believed it was a very bad omen for the year ahead if a piece of mistletoe should fall and touch the earth. Modern Druids might ceremonially touch a branch of cut mistletoe to the earth as a symbol of bringing Heaven to Earth.

Today we have the lovely tradition of kissing under the mistletoe at Christmas. As is so common with the myths involving plants, the story involves a god. The Norse god Balder was known as the Shining God because he was so beautiful, but he was plagued by dreams that predicted he was to die. All the gods and goddesses loved Balder, so they extracted a promise from every living creature that it would not harm Balder. Because he was immune from harm, the gods enjoyed a game of throwing missiles at the beautiful god (which would always miss him). Of course, the beloved one had a jealous enemy who, upon feigning concern that nothing could harm him, found out that there was one small and insignificant tree, mistletoe, which had not been asked to help because it was considered to be too small and weak to be capable of harming Balder anyway. But as the years passed, the small tree grew larger and stronger. The jealous god cut a length from its branches to make a powerful arrow which he tricked Balder's blind brother into throwing at Balder, killing him. The gods were so distraught that mistletoe was uprooted and placed high up on a tree where it could do no harm. It was also decreed that whosoever walks beneath the mistletoe should kiss, to show that this is a plant of love, not hate.

The Magic of the Hedgerow

Plant medicine and wild things have always been associated with magic. The indigenous people of all lands hold deep reverence for certain trees, mountaintops, lakes, springs, plants and animals. Not all that long ago the people of the British Isles absolutely believed that the faery race inhabited the land. Old books relate stories about encounters with 'the Good Folk' who were not the diminutive winged creatures at all. It seems that as the Victorians were steaming ahead scientifically, they sought to trivialise embarrassing old beliefs of the wise women of the village, or the fair folk, or anything that represented primitive ways of thinking. The old understanding of faerie was that these beings were of human size, or maybe taller, or maybe smaller, often of fine features, very powerful and not always nice. They could be mischievous or downright nasty and village folk went out of their way to placate the faeries. The Anglo-Saxons regarded elves with great respect and trepidation, with many spells devised to offset their elven magic.

Spells to counter elven or faerie magic invariably included herbs, as this account written in 1628 shows. "...the women are most frequently to be seen by moonshine: then they dance their rounds in the high grass... It is also necessary to watch cattle that they may not graze in any place where the Elle-people [elves] have been; for if any animal come to a place where the Elle-people have spit or done what is worse, it is attacked by some grievous disease, which can only be cured by giving it to eat a handful of St John's wort, which had been pulled at twelve o'clock on St John's night."

The Ogham Tree Alphabet

By far less well known than the Nordic runes, the Celtic Ogham is an ancient Irish alphabet dating from around 2,000 years ago. One theory suggests that it may have been developed by the Druids as a secret method of communication during the time of the Roman resistance. However, Ogham has also been inscribed on stones for more mundane reasons such as boundary markers or graves. There are ancient examples carved on standing stones in Devon, Cornwall, Wales, the Isle of Man, Scotland and Shetland, but the richest source of ancient Ogham inscriptions are found in Ireland. Short messages were probably inscribed onto wooden staves but these will have perished long ago.

Our current understanding is that the names of the twenty main letters correspond with the names and symbolic meanings of the twenty trees most sacred to the Druids. Each tree has a specific meaning, thus so do the Ogham letters. These symbols can readily be found online.

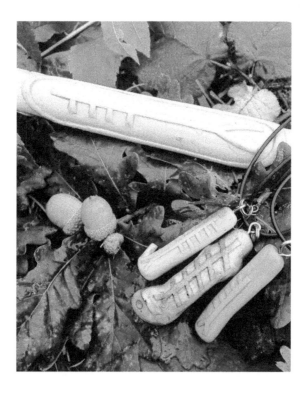

Sometimes called the Celtic Tree Alphabet, people do write messages to each other in Ogham today and the symbols are worn as talismans, but it is mainly used as a method of divination, tapping into the wisdom of the trees. For example, suppose you are wondering whether your relationship is going to survive and you draw the elder. This may suggest the end of a cycle but that a new cycle of your life will come along in time. Once you have accepted that there is no hope of saving the relationship, you may choose to wear birch as a talisman, in order to connect with the energy of sweeping out old energies and bringing a fresh start into your life. You may choose to spend time under a birch in meditation, where you can be refreshed and ready for a new aspect of your life to be born.

The Meanings of the Trees

Beith (Birch)

New beginnings, a fresh start or clean sweep; cleansing, detoxification.

Luis (Rowan)

Protection against chaos or others' harmful intentions (for example, law suits or psychic attack).

Fern (Alder)

Endurance and strength, protection and nurturing. A time to trust one's own instincts.

Nuinn (Ash)

Connections on many levels: the past, present and future, and between the microcosm and macrocosm, bringing universal understanding and awareness of cause and effect.

Saille (Willow)

Inspiring imagination and creativity, strengthening the intuition; also helping us to let go and surrender to the flow of life.

Huath (Hawthorn)

The tree of the heart, love on all levels: the union of the god and the goddess, of man and woman. Protection. The Faery tree.

Duir (Oak)

Strength, stability, security and endurance; a doorway to our inner spirituality and to greater wisdom.

Tinne (Holly)

The protective love that one has for family; this gives direction and willingness to fight for a just cause.

Coll (Hazel)

Creativity and wisdom, inspired by the divine.

Quert (Apple)

Beauty, healing and regeneration; youth and love. Journeying to the Land of Faery. Needing to make a choice between two equally beautiful options.

Muin (Blackberrry)

Harvest, generosity, abundance, wealth and merry-making. Letting go of inhibitions.

Gort (Ivy)

Clinging on tenaciously, smothering or feeling smothered; searching for one's own light or self-expression. This symbolises uniting with others or unwinding bonds.

Ngeadal (Broom, Reed, Wheat)

Direct communication, preservation of knowledge.

Straif (Blackthorn)

Fate that cannot be avoided, a dark time ahead, unavoidable strife, chaos. This difficult period cannot be escaped, but blackthorn can form an impenetrable hedge, hiding and protecting us from the worst.

Ruis (Elder)

The continuous turning of the wheel of life. The ending of the old and opening to the new. A time of change, transformation and evolution.

Ailm (Fir or Pine)

Clarity, for seeing things more clearly; giving a bird's eye view of one's life or of the events in life. The purification of one's body, mind and spirit.

Onn (Gorse)

Bringing home the honey, both in terms of wisdom and a reward for hard work. A light at the end of the tunnel; good things coming our way. A quest achieved. Courage.

Ur (Heather)

The sweetness of life, love and community. Joy. Guidance from the spirit world.

Eadha (Poplar, Aspen)

The ability to hear or see the subtle messages written in our lives. The need to listen to one's inner voice.

Iodhadh (Yew)

Death and renewal. From the darkness comes light, and light returns again to darkness. Nothing lasts forever.

January

There really isn't much to see and do in the hedgerows at this time of the year, but it is a marvellous opportunity to toast our toes near the fire and tell magical hedgerow stories. In our sophisticated society, most people snort at the whimsical stories of plants and faery beings, but I often find that there is some information based on historical fact, or that is part fact and part legend. The tale of The Physicians of Myddfai represents such a story.

A poor widow sends her son to graze the cows at the side of a lake called Llun Y Fan Fach. The lad wanders along the lake and is amazed as his eyes fall upon the most beautiful maiden he has ever seen; she is sitting on top of the lake, combing her hair. Of course, he falls instantly in love and offers her some of his bread. Eventually she glides over but dismisses his bread as being too hard-baked. He rushes home to tell his mother about his beloved. She has an inkling what this is about and suggests that he takes soft white dough instead. All the next day he loiters along the lake edge and just as it is getting dark she reappears, but rejects his bread as being too heavy. That night, the mother half-bakes the bread and her son goes back the following day to offer the lady his softer bread. To the young man's joy, she accepts his bread and his offer of marriage. Just then she disappears into the lake and reappears with an identical twin sister and an old man, her father.

The old man agrees to the marriage only if the groom can tell which sister is his fiancé. Both maidens look exactly alike, but one furtively pushes her foot forward and the young man claims her as the one. The old man claps his hand and says she may marry him and take as many cows, sheep, horses and goats as she can count in one breath. Cleverly she counts in fives and a long line of animals follow the couple to the mother's home. But there is, naturally, a condition. If the husband should ever strike his wife three times, she will return to the lake forever.

They live very happily for many years, producing fine sons, but one day he taps her sharply once for crying loudly at a wedding. She looks at him and says, "That is the first strike." Years pass and then one day she forgets his gloves as they are leaving home and he gently slaps her bottom. "Be careful husband, for that is the second strike."

One day they are attending a funeral when she laughs out loud. The man taps her on the shoulder and says, "Wife, this is not seemly. Why are you laughing at this funeral?" She answers that she laughed because the troubles of the dead are over now, but his are just beginning... and with that, she walks away towards the lake. Following her are all the animals who came with her dowry and no matter how fast her husband and sons run, they cannot catch her. She walks into the lake and disappears beneath the surface.

Her husband never saw her again, but her sons also grieved their mother and she would sometimes appear to them when their father was not about. She taught them how to heal with herbs and told them that they would be the most famous physicians in the land, which indeed they became. For many generations, the Physicians of Myddfai were healers to the kings of Europe as well as to the peasants. They were first recorded in the 12th century and the lineage continued until 1739 when John Jones, the last of them, died. Today, near Llandovery in Carmarthenshire, Wales, there is a museum dedicated to the Physicians of Myddfai and the lady of the lake.

The Birch Tree (*Betula alba*)

The elegant birch is known by some as the White Lady of the Woods and, truly, if you have ever had the joy of walking in the woods on a glittering frosty night under a full moon, you might have come across a grove of silvery birch trees swaying gently like the dancers of Swan Lake. Just like the graceful willow, the fluidity of its movement gives a clue to the plant's therapeutic properties.

Birch is rich in salicylates, the natural constituent found in white willow and meadowsweet from which aspirin is derived, and this accounts for its traditional use in treating pain and stiffness in the joints. In natural medicine, we acknowledge that arthritis is the result of wear and tear on the cartilage, but we also find that through poor diet toxins accumulate in the joints and form crystalline structures. These sharp-edged crystals irritate the joint membranes, causing inflammation, but by stimulating the body to flush out the crystals, pain can be much relieved.

Birch offers a triple remedy when it comes to arthritic conditions. The aspirin-like salicylates in the sap relieve the inflammation and pain, whilst the plant also acts as a kidney tonic, stimulating the flushing out of toxic crystals in the urine. By stimulating the kidneys, water retention is also reduced, and this can help to ease the weight on the joints. Those who hobble about stiffly from creaky, swollen joints may find that by drinking birch leaf tea two or three times a day they may regain at least some of their grace of movement.

Birch is the original spring tonic. Early in the year, before the leaf bud breaks open, the sap begins to rise. This is the life force of the plant rising up again after the long winter spent hibernating deep within the earth. Now the upward rising forces of spring draw the sap towards the light. For a long time, people have tapped the birch sap and drunk it as a spring tonic to cleanse the blood. The idea of the tonic was to imbibe the life-giving forces captured within the birch sap, thus bringing renewed vigour to the human being after the long cold months of meat and wrinkled root vegetables.

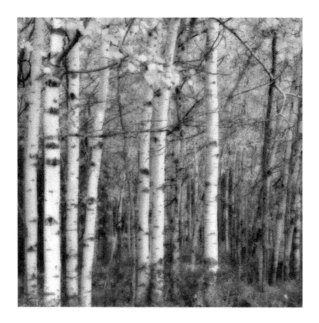

The tree has been used not only for its biological detoxifying properties, but also magically as a besom for hundreds or possibly thousands of years to symbolically sweep out old stagnant energies, thus allowing for new beginnings. Modern Druids might use a birch wand or wear a birch pendant as a talisman to facilitate a new start and welcome in fresh changes in their lives or circumstances. For instance, if you are starting a new business or moving into a new house, or welcoming a new relationship, you might use a birch wand in your ceremony or wear a birch pendant. In older times, the birch stick was also used to whip naughty children, driving out the evil spirits which caused them to be disobedient!

In Germany, there was an old custom that if a man wanted to marry a lady, he would plant a birch tree in her garden and, in that way, they were betrothed. Modern Germans emphasise that she had to marry him and he did not need to ask her. If he planted the birch tree, they were in a sealed contract. They also say darkly that if you happened to hate someone, one option of vengeance was to arrange for a dislikeable man to plant a birch in her garden...

The Pine Tree (*Pinus sylvestris*)

Observe the tall pine, standing high on the mountains with its single trunk pointing straight up towards the clear sky. The pine represents purity. It stands high in the clear mountain air, way above the cares of we mortals in the towns, purifying the air at the same time with its glorious fragrance. The fragrance of pine comes from the oils within the needles and sap, and this essential oil is very antibiotic, purifying the body from infection.

The French have a delicious tradition of boiling young pine buds in sugar and water to extract pine syrup. This is bottled for winter coughs and chest infections, and I am told that children will sometimes feign a cough just to have a mouthful of this tasty syrup. The needles disinfect the lungs and stimulate expectoration of thick sticky phlegm. The medicinal value of the plant is to purify the lungs.

In England, there is a different tradition where the essential oil is used as a rubbing agent to stimulate blood flow to aching muscles and joints. There are several scientific studies that demonstrate the remarkable anti-inflammatory and wound-healing properties of pine essential oils.

When I was a child in South Africa, we used to collect the sticky resin from wounds in the pine trees and use it to glue flowers and feathers onto pieces of bark, producing our own little rustic master-pieces. And the resin would get everywhere, especially on bare sunburnt legs, making bath time a painful affair of picking off the resin which had glued securely to the hairs on our legs. I still love to collect the dried resin from the bark of pine trees and particularly enjoy throwing these crystals onto glowing coals. Immediately, cathedral-like incense is released into the air, bringing the beauty of the pine forest right into my home. I cannot confirm this, but I have an instinct that pine resin has been used for purification rituals for thousands of years.

It is an absolute treat to make oneself bath salts with pine and Siberian fir essential oils. Combined, these oils have the ability to relax the mind and re-invigorate the body. They are absolutely perfect after a very busy week in winter, when one can lie back in the bath with candles alight and float in the warm water with the refreshing fragrance of pine and pure high mountain air. The oils are particularly helpful for those who feel they have negative energy attached to their psychic fields: the pine dispels this energy, purifying the energy fields and invigorating one's whole being.

Pine and Fir Bath Salts

1 cupful of Epsom salts
10 drops of pine essential oil
10 drops of Siberian fir essential oil
2 drops of lavender essential oil

Mix these together and toss them into a hot bath. Do make sure that you drink plenty of cool water while you sink into bliss.

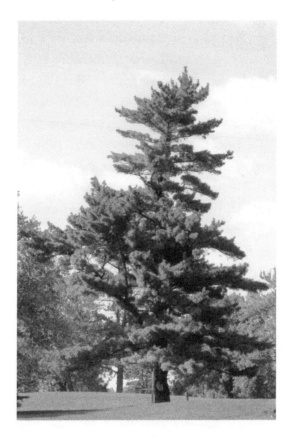

Greater Periwinkle (*Vinca major*)

Periwinkle is used a great deal on roadside islands as an attractive but tough ground cover, even though they would far prefer to be growing under the moist, gentle shade of a forest. Such is the shame of modern living, because this now demoted roadside plant was a deeply respected herb in faraway herbal history. For hundreds of years, it was valued as a protective herb against 'wykked spirytis', against venomous beasts, possessions by demons or envy, and as such was known as the Sorcerer's Violet. The Lucnunga Manuscript tells us, "This wort is of good advantage for many purposes, that is to say first against devil sickness and demoniacal possessions and against snakes and wild beasts and against poisons and for various wishes and for envy and for terror and that thou mayst have grace, and if thou hast the wort with thee thou shalt be prosperous and ever acceptable."

It goes on to give detailed instructions as to how the plant should be harvested. "This wort thou shalt pluck thus, saying, 'I pray thee, Vinca pervinca, thee that art to be had for thy many useful qualities, that thou come to me glad blossoming with thy mainfulness, that thou outfit me so that I be shielded and ever prosperous and undamaged by poisons and by water'; when thou shalt pluck this wort thou shalt be clean of every uncleanness, and thou shalt pick it when the moon is nine nights old and eleven nights and thirteen nights and thirty nights and when it is one night old."

It was used by the local wise folk as part of a love potion, being ground into a powder along with most unfortunate earthworms. This potion was said to keep a husband and wife in love with one another if it was added to their food, probably because of the intertwining actions of the worms and the weed.

These days we use periwinkle for much more mundane purposes. The herb has a relaxing antispasmodic action and has a particular effect on the cerebral arteries, opening the blood flow to the brain and working in a similar manner to Gingko biloba, except that it does not thin the blood as Gingko does. By relaxing the mind and gently dilating the blood vessels, this herb helps to reduce blood pressure and improves memory at the same time. Why would we use Gingko imported from China when we have this alternative growing right in our own gardens?

Periwinkle is also an astringent herb, effective against diarrhoea, sore throats and heavy periods. For less mundane purposes, it is said to be useful in alleviating 'lunacy' – for those many people who feel that the energies of the full moon disrupt their sense of balance and mood. I have a patient who tells me that she is a 'lunatic', and goes to great lengths to avoid finding out when the moon is full as she just cannot sleep and becomes quite bad-mannered. I asked if she would like to try some *Vinca* and she reported back later that it had helped her to feel calmer.

Who is The Green Man?

Before the Romans invaded Britain 2,000 years ago and beyond, the Druids were the priests of these islands. They practised their ceremonies within circular groves of trees deep in the forests, for their holy place was outside in nature, under the leafy roof of their gods and goddesses.

To break the power of the Druids, the Romans began to cut down their sacred groves. This caused so much anguish to the Druids, who for generations had venerated the trees of their groves, that they chose to cut the trees themselves so that the destruction was done with mourning, grief and honour. Later, as churches and cathedrals started to rise, the stonemasons, who may still have had roots in the Old Religion, carved stone forests of towering arches. High up near the ceiling, within the stone greenery, the faces of Green Men peer down at the congregation below. Their strange faces burst out of the greenery with foliage sprouting from their mouths and eyes, for they embodied the spirit of nature, the god of the wilderness. Why they were placed in the churches is unknown, but perhaps the masons did not want the spirit of the greenwood to be forgotten or lost in the new Christian religion.

As it happens, the Green Man survived in many guises: he morphed into Robin Hood who lived among the trees, he was sung as Jack-in-the-Green and he is remembered during the May games. His spirit is everywhere, and now ever more in our consciousness as nature-honouring spiritual beliefs grow in popularity in conjunction with the political Green movement.

The Green Man is symbolic of the god of the woodland, or the voice of nature, that life spirit which enlivens the forest with the sense of intelligence and magic. His green mantle covers the goddess who is the Earth. If you are sensitive to feeling this lightness of spirit or a quickening of power when you step among the greenery, it may be that you are feeling the Green Man near you.

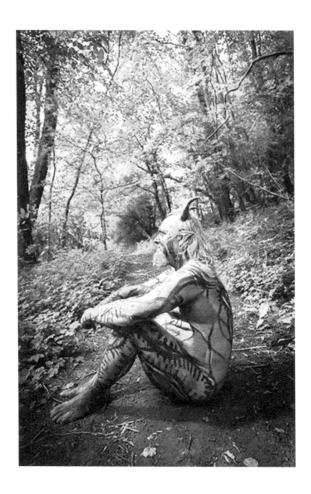

References

Lichens

(1) Antimicrobial and antibiofilm activity of secondary metabolites of lichens against methicillin-resistant Staphylococcus aureus strains from cystic fibrosis patients. Pompilio AI, Pomponio S, Di Vincenzo V, Crocetta V, Nicoletti M, Piovano M, Garbarino JA, Di Bonaventura G. (Future Microbiol. 2013 Feb; 8(2): 281-92. doi: 10.2217/fmb.12.142.)

(2) Potent activity of the lichen antibiotic (+)-usnic acid against clinical isolates of vancomycin-resistant enterococci and methicillin-resistant Staphylococcus aureus. Elo HI, Matikainen J, Pelttari E. (Naturwissenschaften. 2007 Jun; 94(6): 465-8. Epub 2007 Jan 24.)

(3) The antimicrobial activity of extracts of the lichen Cladonia foliacea and its (-)-usnic acid, atranorin, and fumarprotocetraric acid constituents. Yilmaz MI, Türk AO, Tay T, Kivanç M. (Z Naturforsch C. 2004 Mar-Apr; 59(3-4): 249-54.)

(4) Antimycobacterial activity of lichen substances. Honda NKI, Pavan FR, Coelho RG, de Andrade Leite SR, Micheletti AC, Lopes TI, Misutsu MY, Beatriz A, Brum RL, (Leite Phytomedicine. 2010 Apr; 17(5): 328-32. doi: 10.1016/j.phymed.2009.07.018. Epub 2009 Aug 14.CQ.)

(5) Activity of Scottish plant, lichen and fungal endophyte extracts against mycobacterium aurum and mycobacterium tuberculosis. Gordien AYI, Gray AI, Ingleby K, Franzblau SG, Seidel V. (Phytother Res. 2010 May; 24(5): 692-8. doi: 10.1002/ptr.2988.)

(6) Antimicrobial activity of extracts of the lichen Parmelia sulcata and its salazinic acid constituent. Candan MI, Yilmaz M, Tay T, Erdem M, Türk AO. (Z Naturforsch C. 2007 Jul-Aug; 62(7-8): 619-21.)

Sphagnum Moss
(7) Biological properties of the Chilean native moss Sphagnum magellanicum. Montenegro GI, Portaluppi MC, Salas FA, Díaz MF. (Biol Res. 2009; 42(2): 233-7. doi: /S0716-97602009000200012. Epub 2009 Aug 20.)

Wild Garlic
(8) Wild garlic has a greater effect than regular garlic on blood pressure and blood chemistries of rats. Preuss HGI, Clouatre D, Mohamadi A, Jarrell ST. (Int Urol Nephrol. 2001; 32(4): 525-30.)

Goutweed
(9) Study of the composition of the goutweed flowers essential oil, its renal effects and influence on uric acid exchange. O. Koyro, O.V. Tovchiga, S. I. Stepanova, S. Yu. Shtrygol. (Pharmacognosy Communications, Volume 2 | Issue 3 | Jul-Sep 2012.)

St John's Wort
(10) Identification of light-independent inhibition of human immunodeficiency virus-I infection through bioguided fractionation of Hypericum perforatum. Maury WI, Price JP, Brindley MA, Oh C, Neighbors JD, Wiemer DF, Wills N, Carpenter S, Hauck C, Murphy P, Widrlechner MP, Delate K, Kumar G, Kraus GA, Rizshsky L, Nikolau B. (Virol J. 2009 Jul 13; 6:101. doi: 10.1186/1743-422X-6-101.)

(11) Inactivation of the human immunodeficiency virus by hypericin: evidence for photochemical alterations of p24 and a block in uncoating. Degar SI, Prince AM, Pascual D, Lavie G, Levin B, Mazur Y, Lavie D, Ehrlich LS, Carter C, Meruelo D. (AIDS Res Hum Retroviruses. 1992 Nov; 8(11): 1929-36.)

Elderberry

(12) Anti-influenza virus effects of elderberry juice and its fractions. Kinoshita EI, Hayashi K, Katayama H, Hayashi T, Obata A. (Biosci Biotechnol Biochem. 2012; 76(9): 1633-8. Epub 2012 Sep 7.)

(13) Randomized study of the efficacy and safety of oral elderberry extract in the treatment of influenza A and B virus infections. Zakay-Rones ZI, Thom E, Wollan T, Wadstein J. (J Int Med Res. 2004 Mar-Apr; 32(2): 132-40.)

(14) Virus susceptibility and clinical effectiveness of anti-influenza drugs during the 2010-2011 influenza season in Russia. Leneva IAI, Burtseva EI2, Yatsyshina SB3, Fedyakina IT2, Kirillova ES2, Selkova EP4, Osipova E5, Maleev VV3. (Int J Infect Dis. 2016 Feb; 43: 77-84. doi: 10.1016/j.ijid.2016.01.001.)

Mugwort

(15) Antimicrobial activity of Artemisia vulgaris LINN. (Damanaka). Hiremath SK, Kolume DG, Muddapur UM. (IJRAP 2011, 2 (6) 1674-1675.)

(16) Antimalarial properties of Artemisia vulgaris L. ethanolic leaf extract in a plasmodium berghei murine malaria model. Bamunuarachchi GS, Ratnasooriya WD, Premakumara S, Udagama PV. (J Vector Borne Dis. 2013 Dec; 50(4): 278-84.)

(17) In-vitro cytotoxicity of Artemisia vulgaris L. essential oil is mediated by a mitochondria-dependent apoptosis in HL-60 leukemic cell line. Saleh AMI, Aljada A, Rizvi SA, Nasr A, Alaskar AS, Williams JD. (BMC Complement Altern Med. 2014 Jul 7; 14:226. doi: 10.1186/1472-6882-14-226.)

(18) Anticancer activity of Artemisia vulgaris on hepatocellular carcinoma (HEPG2) cells. Sharmilla K, Padma PR. (International Journal of Pharmacy and Pharmaceutical Sciences Vol 5, Suppl 3, 2013)

(19) The Quest for Cognition in Plant Neurobiology. Francisco Calvo Garzón. (Plant Signal Behav. 2007 Jul-Aug; 2(4): 208–211.)

Honeysuckle
(20) Honeysuckle-encoded atypical microRNA2911 directly targets influenza A viruses. Zhen Zhou et al. (Cell Research, published online October 07, 2014; doi: 10.1038/cr.2014.130)

Hemp Agrimony
(21) Cytotoxicity of Eupatorium cannabinum L. ethanolic extract against colon cancer cells and interactions with Bisphenol A and Doxorubicin. Ribeiro-Varandas E, Ressurreição F, Viegas W, Delgado M. (BMC Complement Altern Med. 2014 Jul 24; 14:264. doi: 10.1186/1472-6882-14-264.)

Angelica
(22) Essential oil composition and antimicrobial activity of Angelica archangelica L. (apiaceae) roots. Fraternale DI, Flamini G, Ricci D. (J Med Food. 2014 Sep; 17(9): 1043-7.)

(23) Effect of ferulic acid and Angelica archangelica extract on behavioral and psychological symptoms of dementia in frontotemporal lobar degeneration and dementia with Lewy bodies. Kimura TI, Hayashida H, Murata M, Takamatsu J. (Geriatr Gerontol Int. 2011 Jul; 11(3): 309-14.)

(24) Evaluation of antiseizure activity of essential oil from roots of Angelica archangelica linn. in mice. Pathak SI, Wanjari MM, Jain SK, Tripathi M. (Indian J Pharm Sci. 2010 May; 72(3): 371-5.)

(25) Time-course and dose-response relationships of Imperatorin in the mouse maximal electroshock seizure threshold model. Luszczki JJI, Glowniak K, Czuczwar SJ. (Neurosci Res. 2007 Sep; 59(1): 18-22.)

(26) Antiproliferative effect of Angelica archangelica fruits. Sigurdsson SI, Ogmundsdottir HM, Gudbjarnason S. (Z Naturforsch C. 2004 Jul-Aug; 59(7-8): 523-7.)

(27) Antitumour activity of Angelica archangelica leaf extract. Sigurdsson SI, Ogmundsdottir HM, Hallgrimsson J, Gudbjarnason S. (In Vivo. 2005 Jan-Feb; 19(1): 191-4.)

Mistletoe

(28) An exploratory study on the quality of life and individual coping of cancer patients during mistletoe therapy. Brandenberger MI, Simões-Wüst AP, Rostock M, Rist L, Saller R. (Integr Cancer Ther. 2012 Jun; 11(2): 90-100.)

(29) Interaction of standardized mistletoe (Viscum album) extracts with chemotherapeutic drugs regarding cytostatic and cytotoxic effects in-vitro. Ulrike Weissenstein, corresponding author I, Matthias Kunz, I Konrad Urech, I and Stephan Baumgartner. (BMC Complement Altern Med. 2014; 14: 6.)

(30) Adjuvant cancer biotherapy by Viscum album extract isorel: overview of evidence-based medicine findings. Sunjic SB, Gasparovic AC, Vukovic T, Weiss T, Weiss ES, Soldo I, Djakovic N, Zarkovic T, Zarkovic N. (Coll Antropol. 2015 Sep; 39(3): 701-8.)

(31) Clinical evaluation of Viscum album mother tincture as an antihypertensive: a pilot study. Poruthukaren KJI, Palatty PL, Baliga MS, Suresh S. (J Evid Based Complementary Altern Med. 2014 Jan; 19(1): 31-5.)

(32) Vasodilator activity of the aqueous extract of Viscum album. Tenorio FAI, del Valle L, González A, Pastelín G. (Fitoterapia. 2005 Mar; 76(2): 204-9.)

Bibliography

Aloysius, Brother	A Healer's Herbal (Samuel Weiser, 1998)
Bates, Brian	The Real Middle Earth (Sidgwick & Jackson, 2002)
Beith, Mary	Healing Threads (Birlinn Ltd, 1995)
Breverton, Terry	The Physicians of Myddfai (Cambria Books, 2012)
Chamberlain, Mary	Old Wives Tales (Tempus Publishing Ltd, 2006)
Conway, David	The Magic of Herbs (Jonathan Cape, 1973)
Culpeper, Nicolas	Culpeper's Complete Herbal (Wordsworth Editions Ltd, 1995)
DerMarderosian, A	Folk Remedies Healing Wisdom (Publications International Ltd, 1999)
Evans-Wentz, W Y	The Fairy Faith in Celtic Countries (The Lost Libreary, 1911)
Gerard, John	Gerard's Herbal (Studio Editions, 1990)
Gordon, Lesley	A Country Herbal (Webb & Bower, 1980)
Grieve, M	A Modern Herbal (Penguin Books, 1980)
Hageneder, Fred	The Spirits of Trees (Floris Books, 2006)
Hatfield, Gabrielle	Hatfield's Herbal (Allen Lane, 2007)
Hoffmann, David	Welsh Herbal Medicine (Abercastle Publications, 2007)

Mabey, Richard   Flora Britannica (Chatto & Windus, 1996)

Matthews, John   The Quest for the Green Man (Godsfield Press, 2001)

Matthews, John   The Secret Lives of Elves & Faeries (Godsfield Press, 2005)

Michell, John   New Light on the Ancient Mystery of Glastonbury (Gothic Image Publications, 1997)

Miles, David   The Tribes of Britain (Phoenix, 2006)

Phillips, Roger   Wild Flowers of Britain (Pan Books, 1977)

Phillips, Roger   Wild Food (Pan Books, 1983)

Popescu, Charlotte   Fruits of the Hedgerow and Unusual Garden Fruits (Cavalier Paperbacks, 2011)

Price, Dennis   The Missing Years of Jesus (Hay House, 2009)

Ramsbottom John   Mushrooms and Toadstools (Collins, 1953)

Rawcliffe, Carole   Medicine & Society in Later Medieval England (Sandpiper Books, 1999)

Schofield, Bernard   A Miscellany of Garden Wisdom (HarperCollins, 1996)

Tarrant, Tina   What's Your Poison? (Capall Bann Publishing, 2004)

Vickery, Roy   A Dictionary of Plant Lore (Oxford University Press, 1995)

Wren, R C   Potter's New Cyclopaedia of Botanical Drugs and Preparations (The C W Daniel Company Limited, 1985)

Resources

The Order of Bards, Ovates and Druids

www.druidry.org
OBOD, PO Box 1333, Lewes, East Sussex, BN7 IDX
T. 01273 470888 ; E. office@druidry.org

The British Druid Order

www.druidry.co.uk

The National Institute of Medical Herbalists

Clover House, James Court, South Street, Exeter, EXI IEE
T. 01392 426022 ; www.nimh.org.uk ; E. info@nimh.org.uk

The College of Practitioners of Phytotherapy

Pam Bull, CPP, Oak Glade, 9 Hythe Close,
Polegate, East Sussex, BN26 6LQ
T. 01323 484353 ; www.phytotherapists.org ;
E. pamela.bull@phytotherapists.org

Wildways Body Painting Project

www.wildwaysontheborle.co.uk ; E. wildwaysontheborle@gmail.com

Adrian Rooke

Pagan celebrant, Ogham pendants and wands, spiritual counselling.
E. adeoftheoldways@hotmail.co.uk

Botanica Medica Herbal Apothecary

Jo Dunbar, 24 Crown Rd, St Margaret's,
Twickenham, Middlesex, TW1 3EE
T. 0208 8929227
Jo Dunbar, 5 Sydney Terrace, The Green, Claygate,
Esher, Surrey, KT10 0JJ
T. 01372 470990 ; www.botanicamedica.co.uk ;
E. info@botanicamedica.co.uk

Index of Botanical Names

Achillia millefolium	Yarrow
Aconitum napellus	Aconite, wolfbane
Aegopodium podograria	Ground elder, goutweed
Aesculus hippocastrum	Horse chestnut
Alchemilla vulgaris	Lady's mantle
Allium ursinum	Wild garlic
Alliaria petiolata	Hedge mustard, Jack-by-the-Hedge
Althea officinalis	Marshmallow
Amanita muscaria	Fly agaric
Amoracia rusticana	Horseradish
Angelica archangelica	Angelica
Angelica sylvestris	Alexanders
Arctium lappa	Burdock
Artemisia vulgaris	Mugwort
Bellis perennis	Daisy
Betula alba	Birch
Castanea sativa	Sweet chestnut
Calluna vulgaris	Heather
Capsella bursa pastoris	Shepherd's purse
Chelidonium majus	Greater celandine

Crataegus spp.	Hawthorn, May blossom
Dryopteris filix-mas	Male fern
Equisetum arvense	Horsetail, mare's tail
Eupatorium cannabinum	Hemp agrimony
Filipendula ulmaria	Meadowsweet
Gallium aparine	Cleavers, goosegrass, sticky willy
Glechoma hederacea	Ground ivy
Heracleum mantegazzianum	Hogweed
Humulus lupulus	Hops
Hypericum perfoliatum	St John's wort
Ilex aquifolium	Holly
Inula helenium	Elecampane, elfwort
Lactuca virosa	Wild lettuce
Lamium album	White deadnettle
Lonicera pericymenum	Honeysuckle
Myrica odorata	Sweet cicely
Oenothera biennsis	Evening primrose
Parietaria diffusa	Pellitory-of-the-wall
Papaver rhoes	Field poppy, corn poppy
Pinus sylvestris	Pine tree
Plantago lanceolata	Ribwort
Plantago major	Plantain
Primula veris	Cowslip

Prunus spinosa	Blackthorn, sloe
Prunus insititia	Bullace, wild plum
Ranunculus ficaria	Lesser celandine
Rosa canina	Dog rose
Rubus fruticosus	Blackberry, bramble
Salix alba	White willow
Sambucus nigra	Elder
Scrophularia nodosa	Figwort
Sphagnum cymbifolium	Sphagnum moss
Sorbus aucuparia	Rowan, mountain ash
Stachys betonica	Betony
Stachys sylvatica	Hedge woundwort
Stellaria media	Chickweed
Symphytum officinalis	Comfrey, knitbone
Taxus baccata	Yew
Tilea cordata	Linden blossom, lime blossom
Trifolium pratense	Red clover
Urtica dioica	Nettles
Usnea spp.	Lichen
Valeriana officinalis	Valerian
Verbena officinalis	Vervain
Vinca major	Periwinkle
Viscum album	Mistletoe

Index of Common Names

Garlic mustard, Jack-by-the-Hedge	*Alliaria petiolata*
Ground elder, Jack-jump-about	*Aegopodium podograria*
Ground ivy	*Glechoma hederacea*
Hawthorn, May blossom	*Crataegus spp.*
Heather	*Calluna vulgaris*
Hedge woundwort	*Stachys sylvatica*
Hemp agrimony	*Eupatorium cannabinum*
Hogweed	*Heracleum mantegazzianum*
Honeysuckle	*Lonicera pericymenum*
Holly	*Ilex aquifolium*
Hops	*Humulus lupulus*
Horsetail, mare's tail	*Equisetum arvense*
Horseradish	*Amoracia rusticana*
Horse chestnut	*Aesculus hippocastrum*
Greater periwinkle	*Vinca major*
Lady's mantle	*Alchemilla vulgaris*
Lawn daisy	*Bellis perennis*
Lesser celandine	*Ranunculus ficaria*
Lichen	*Usnea spp.*
Lime tree, linden tree	*Tilea cordata*
Male ferns	*Dryopteris filix-mas*
Marshmallow	*Althea officinalis*
Meadowsweet	*Filipendula ulmaria*

Mistletoe	*Viscum album*
Mugwort	*Artemisia vulgaris*
Nettles	*Urtica dioica*
Pelitory-of-the-wall	*Parietaria diffusa*
Pine	*Pinus sylvestris*
Plantain	*Plantago major*
Red clover	*Trifolium pratense*
Ribwort	*Plantago lanceolata*
Rowan tree, mountain ash	*Sorbus aucuparia*
Shepherds purse	*Capsella bursa pastoris*
Sloes, blackthorn	*Prunus spinosa*
Sphagnum moss	*Sphagnum cymbifolium*
St John's wort	*Hypericum perfoliatum*
Sweet cicely	*Myrica odorata*
Sweet chestnut	*Castanea sativa*
Valerian	*Valeriana officinalis*
Vervain	*Verbena officinalis*
White dead-nettle	*Lamium album*
White willow	*Salix alba*
Wild garlic ransoms	*Allium ursinum*
Wild lettuce	*Lactuca virosa*
Yarrow	*Achillia millefolium*
Yew	*Taxus baccata*

If you have enjoyed this book...

Local Legend is committed to publishing the very best spiritual writing, both fiction and non-fiction. You might also enjoy:

AURA CHILD
A I Kaymen (ISBN 978-1-907203-71-8)

One of the most astonishing books ever written, telling the true story of a genuine Indigo child. Genevieve grew up in a normal London family but from an early age realised that she had very special spiritual and psychic gifts. She saw the energy fields around living things, read people's thoughts and even found herself slipping through time, able to converse with the spirits of those who had lived in her neighbourhood. This is an uplifting and inspiring book for what it tells us about the nature of our minds.

A SINGLE PETAL
Oliver Eade (ISBN 978-1-907203-42-8)

Winner of the first national Local Legend Spiritual Writing Competition, this page-turner is a novel of murder, politics and passion set in ancient China. Yet its themes of loyalty, commitment and deep personal love are every bit as relevant for us today as they were in past times. The author is an expert on Chinese culture and history, and his debut adult novel deserves to become a classic.

A UNIVERSAL GUIDE TO HAPPINESS
Joanne Gregory (ISBN 978-1-910027-06-6)

Joanne is an internationally acclaimed clairaudient medium with a celebrity contact list. Growing up, she ignored her evident psychic abilities, fearful of standing out from others, and even later, despite witnessing miracles daily, her life was difficult. But then she began to learn the difference between the psychic and the spiritual, and her life turned round. This is her spiritual reference handbook – a guide to living happily and successfully in harmony with the energy that created our universe. It is the knowledge and wisdom distilled from a lifetime's experience of working with spirit.

THE QUIRKY MEDIUM
Alison Wynne-Ryder (ISBN 978-1-907203-47-3)

Alison is the co-host of the TV show *Rescue Mediums*, in which she puts herself in real danger to free homes of lost and often malicious spirits. Yet she is a most reluctant medium, afraid of ghosts! This is her amazing and often very funny autobiography, taking us 'back stage' of the television production as well as describing how she came to discover the psychic gifts that have brought her an international following.

Winner of the Silver Medal in the national Wishing Shelf Book Awards.

5PIRIT R3V3L4T10N5
Nigel Peace (ISBN 978-1-907203-14-5)

With descriptions of more than a hundred proven prophetic dreams and many more everyday synchronicities, the author shows us that, without doubt, we can know the future and that everyone can receive genuine spiritual guidance for our lives' challenges. World-renowned biologist Dr Rupert Sheldrake has endorsed this book as "…vivid and fascinating… pioneering research…" and it was national runner-up in The People's Book Prize awards.

RAINBOW CHILD
S L Coyne (ISBN 978-1-907203-92-3)

Beautifully written in language that is alternately lyrical and childlike, this is the story of young Rebekah and the people she discovers as her family settles in a new town far from their familiar home. As dark family secrets begin to unravel, her life takes many turns both delightful and terrifying as the story builds to a tragic and breathless climax that just keeps on going. This book shows us how we look at others who are 'different'. Through the eyes of Rebekah, writing equally with passion and humour, we see the truth of human nature…

These titles are all available as paperbacks and eBooks.
Further details and extracts of these and many
other beautiful books may be seen at
www.local-legend.co.uk

Lightning Source UK Ltd.
Milton Keynes UK
UKHW020955050720
365988UK00009B/521